D1374415

Delivering Excellence
in Health and Social Care

Delivering Excellence in Health and Social Care

Quality, excellence and
performance measurement

Max Moullin

Open University Press
Buckingham • Philadelphia

Open University Press
Celtic Court
22 Ballmoor
Buckingham
MK18 1XW

email: enquiries@openup.co.uk
world wide web: www.openup.co.uk

and

325 Chestnut Street
Philadelphia, PA 19106, USA

First Published 2002

A catalogue record of this book is available from the British Library

ISBN   0 335 20888 6 (pbk)   0 335 20889 4 (hbk)

Library of Congress Cataloging-in-Publication Data
Moullin, Max, 1953–
    Delivering excellence in health and social care: quality, excellence, and
performance measurement/Max Moullin.
        p. cm.
    Includes bibliographical references and index.
    ISBN 0-335-20888-6 (pbk.) – ISBN 0-335-20889-4 (hb)
        1. Medical care–Quality control. 2. Social services. 3. Medical policy. I. Title.

RA394 .M685 2002
362.1'068'5–dc21

                                                                                    2002022792

Typeset by Graphicraft Limited, Hong Kong
Printed in Great Britain by Biddles Limited, Guildford and King's Lynn

Contents

Foreword

My position fortunately affords me the opportunity to visit a great many NHS organizations and to speak with both front-line staff and patients. In the course of these visits, I invariably ask everyone I meet to tell me of their greatest concern or worry in relation to the NHS. Although the reply is expressed in a variety of ways, there is inevitably a common theme. For staff it will be to ensure that we are always providing the best possible 'quality' care for our patients, and for the patients themselves it will be that they always receive the highest standard of care and treatment.

It is without doubt true that quality matters. That conclusion leads us on to a whole new set of questions. What do we really mean by a quality service? Is it seen differently by those who provide the services and by those patients, clients and citizens for whom the services are provided? Just as importantly, once we know how to measure quality, how can we work to improve it? All too often, busy workers in the caring professions simply don't have the time or the tools to consider these issues properly.

Max Moullin goes a long way towards providing professionals with the kind of insight which they most urgently require. His review of the different approaches to measuring quality and to promoting excellence in health and social care is comprehensive and thorough. Just as importantly, it is rooted in practical reality. His published competitors in this field usually draw heavily upon private sector examples – examples which those working in the NHS, social services and the voluntary sector find hard to relate to their daily experience. Max makes no such mistake. He draws upon his wealth of public sector knowledge to provide an array of interesting and apposite case studies which illuminate his main themes. As a consequence, his book will be useful not only to those who want an academic perspective, but to anyone who is concerned with improving the service they provide.

Following a recent discussion with a group of doctors, one of them said to me, 'Ah, so that's what quality improvement means – well we can do that, I thought it was far more complicated'. I would hope that this is just the kind of reaction that the current volume will evoke. As Max himself says, 'excellence in health and social care is something to which staff, service users, patients and carers all aspire'. This book should undoubtedly help its readers in their pursuit of that aspiration.

David Fillingham
Director of the NHS Modernization Agency

Introduction

Many organizations in health and social care are striving to implement the ideas of organizational excellence, performance measurement and process improvement in the context of a wide variety of government initiatives including the National Health Service (NHS) Plan, Best Value, Clinical Governance and Quality Protects. The aim of this book is to provide clarity in this whole area and to help organizations in health and social care to deliver better quality services for service users, many of whom will be feeling anxious, vulnerable or in pain.

Delivering excellence in health and social care requires commitment from all involved, including government ministers and local councillors, who need to ensure resources are available, and all managers and staff providing a service either directly or indirectly to patients and service users. Commitment is needed to develop a motivated and capable workforce, to partnership working and user involvement, to improving processes and developing new ways of working, and above all to providing improved services to patients, service users and carers. However, commitment alone is not sufficient. People need to learn from others – both in health and social care and elsewhere – to identify best practice and to learn how to apply what they have learnt to their own organizations or departments.

The book is in three parts: quality, excellence, and performance measurement. The first part examines what services should look like from the point of view of patients, carers and other service users. It looks at the relationship between quality and cost and quality and equity, and compares a number of approaches to quality management, referring to the teaching of some acknowledged quality 'gurus' and some of the main quality-related initiatives in health and social care. Finally it examines the relevance of service standards and the international quality standard ISO9000.

Part 2, on excellence, is the heart of the book, covering the use of the Excellence Model together with extensive discussion, advice and case studies on the different enablers of the model – leadership and policy and strategy, people development and involvement, partnerships and user involvement, and process improvement. Part 3, on performance measurement, examines a number of approaches to measuring performance including the balanced scorecard and the performance prism as well as the Excellence Model.

As Professor Mike Pringle (2001) of the Royal College of General Practitioners says, 'We need as a matter of urgency to look at the way in which services are delivered and continue to develop initiatives to promote excellent quality of care'. This book aims to assist in this process.

PART one

Quality

CHAPTER one

What is quality in health and social care?

Why quality?

The vast majority of people working in health and social care are concerned with the quality of the service they provide. Indeed, it is this which motivates them day in and day out in their everyday work which is, in many cases, lower paid and more demanding than that of people in other jobs. However, while the need for quality is perhaps self-evident, it is useful to list some of the main reasons *why* quality is important:

- it is important for patients and service users;
- it is important for staff;
- it can help reduce costs and provide an even better service within a given budget.

Importance for patients and service users

Patients and service users not only benefit directly from quality as their requirements are better met but also indirectly, as the next time they come into contact with a particular service they will feel more confident that they will also be treated well. Patients, service users and their relatives are often worried, anxious, stressed, frightened and vulnerable. Such feelings are exacerbated by long waits, insufficient information, insensitivity to their needs and poor facilities. All that can be done to lessen these feelings and improve the quality of their experience will be well received.

Importance for staff

The majority of staff chose a career in health and social care due to a real desire and commitment to care for people in need, often sacrificing opportunities for more money or more convenient working hours. Where the service is not organized properly staff find it difficult to provide the level of care and concern that they wish to give and they become demotivated and frustrated.

A well-designed quality improvement programme empowering staff to decide what can be done and then supporting them in their efforts to improve quality is a way out of this spiral. The benefits to staff are likely to include increased job satisfaction, less frustration as other groups of staff improve their quality, better feedback from patients and service users and greater self-worth, as the reputation of their department or unit improves.

Importance for reducing costs

There is of course a strong relationship between quality and the resources provided. There can be no substitute for additional social workers, support workers, nurses, doctors, information technology (IT) staff, porters and other staff. Indeed, as the National Institute for Social Work (2001) says, many service users cannot see how quality can be improved without addressing fundamental issues like resources.

However, investing in quality services can, like any other investment, reduce costs. There are two main ways in which this occurs. First, better quality services can reduce the costs associated with poor quality. For example, if a surgical operation does not go well there may be no opportunity to put it right. Similarly if a child is placed in the care of an unsuitable foster carer, there can be very substantial costs to the child in terms of their social and emotional development, together with additional costs to the social services department which will then have to spend a great deal of time finding a more suitable placement. As Carruthers and Holland (1991) put it, 'Good quality may not always save money, but poor quality always costs and usually wastes money'.

In many cases, quality improvements will increase the costs for one department or organization while reducing costs elsewhere. For example, better discharge arrangements by social workers may reduce the costs of patient stays in hospital, while investing in better quality services for looked-after children may not only reduce social services costs in future years, but also produce considerable savings for the criminal justice system. There needs to be a mechanism for investing in one area to achieve savings elsewhere.

The other way that improving quality can reduce costs is based on the fact that many costs incurred in running a service add little value to service users and in fact cause unnecessary delays. For example, an over-complicated procedure for referring patients to a particular clinic would lead to both additional costs and longer waiting times for patients. Redesigning the referral process to eliminate activities that do not add value would both reduce costs and improve quality.

Implications of poor quality in a hospital

Table 1.1 illustrates the implications of certain recurrent quality problems in a hospital, and shows clearly the importance of quality – for patients and service users, for staff and for reducing costs.

Approaches to defining quality

Managers in health and social care are under considerable pressure to improve the quality of their services. But what exactly does 'quality' mean? As Gaster (1995) says, 'Definitions are important: they drive the whole implementation process and are the basis of standard setting and measurement'. Whenever difficulties arrive in implementation, a clear definition is needed to remind people of what quality is really about. In fact, there is a plethora of different definitions of quality in current use. Reeves and Bednar (1994) have noted this: 'new definitions have not replaced old ones; rather all of the quality definitions continue to be used today'.

The problem is not just the number of definitions in current use, but that many of these definitions give very different messages to managers about what quality really means. Crosby (1992) criticized the Malcolm Baldridge National Quality Award in the USA saying 'there is no definition of quality involved, yet everyone talks "quality" like there's a common understanding'. Crosby's statement is borne out by a survey of quality managers and quality directors carried out by the author (Moullin 1997). Of the survey's 60 respondents, 35 said their organization used a definition of quality in their quality programme. Each of these 35 organizations used a different definition of quality!

This applies similarly to health and social care. As Joss and Kogan (1995) say, 'it would be a mistake to assume that [the drive for quality] is underpinned by common understandings of quality either within the NHS or between the NHS and other organisations. Within the NHS definitions of quality vary profoundly between different groups of staff and between staff and patients'.

There are many ways of defining quality and these are perhaps best examined using the five approaches identified by Garvin (1984). These are discussed in turn below. Examples of definitions in each of the five categories

Table 1.1   Implications of poor quality in a hospital

Description	Implications for patients	Implications for staff	Cost implications
Inadequate clinical details given to pathology department	Delays to patients Risks of incorrect tests	Extra work for pathology staff Extra conversations with clinical customers	Extra pathology costs Increased length of stay Fewer patients treated More complaints Some appointments cancelled
Porters not available to move patients to operating theatre	Delays in operations Sicker patients Patients in for longer	Staff kept waiting Delays in operations Inter-staff aggravation	Expensive staff and plant underused More costly treatments for patients' worsened conditions Higher accommodation costs
Insufficient car parking facilities	Patients late for appointments Increased anxiety	Staff late for appointments Low morale	Staff (or patients) kept waiting Capital equipment not used to fullest capacity Repeated appointments
Health records missing or out of date	Frustration at having to repeat history Wrong treatment offered	Histories need taking again Internal inquiries	Extra time spent searching or taking histories Extra consultations Expensive/complex remedial treatments
Discharge delayed because drugs to take home are not available	Longer stay Longer waits for new patients	Unnecessary work for all staff	Higher accommodation costs Slower throughput
Patients kept waiting over an hour for pre-booked appointments	Stress and frustration Can't park as car parks over-full	Ambulances held up Staff on the defensive	Extra staff time on explaining and mollifying Need for larger waiting rooms and car parks

are shown in Table 1.2 on the diagonal (in italics). Some 'hybrid' definitions containing elements of two different categories are also shown, but they will be examined later.

Transcendent

The transcendent approach dates from the time of Plato and Aristotle and is still the one in most common everyday use outside of business. Quality is seen as the degree of excellence or superiority, often associated with premium products and services like a Rolls-Royce car or the Savoy Hotel.

There are however a number of problems with this approach from a management perspective. For example, while it may provide a clear lead to organizations in premium markets, it is not so relevant to those making a Fiat or to a small guest-house. They will never be able to provide all the features of a Rolls-Royce or the Savoy. Does that mean that they can never aspire towards quality? Does quality not have a meaning for them too?

A second problem with this approach is that it often leads an organization to focus on just some parts of the service they provide. A manufacturing company may concentrate on product rather than service aspects, while health services may concentrate on the excellence of the surgery performed, with little attention to the number of months patients have to wait before they receive the surgery, conditions and queues in the waiting room, and providing appropriate information, guidance and reassurance.

Product-based

Product-based definitions are epitomized by a carpet retailer who asked a customer, 'What width do you want?' and 'What quality do you want?' in successive sentences. Quality was seen as equivalent to the thickness of the pile. However, the customer's requirements, like most people's, included many other factors – the pattern, colour and availability to mention just a few. Such definitions suggest that quality is uni-dimensional and that higher quality must of necessity cost more money.

Another example is the coal industry, where the term 'coal quality' typically refers to its ash content or calorific value. In fact, consistency of the coal (i.e. whether the batch is homogeneous or not) is more important to most industrial customers than the actual ash content or calorific value, as they can make adjustments if they know the characteristics of the particular coal shipment. Also important of course is continuity of supply and a host of other factors.

Manufacturing-based

Manufacturing-based definitions such as conformance to specifications have had a considerable impact on improving quality in the manufacturing

Table 1.2 Pure and hybrid definitions of quality

	Transcendent	Product	Manufacturing	Consumer	Value
Transcendent	*Even though quality cannot be defined, you know what it is* (Pirsig 1974)				
Product	Quality is a principle that encourages excellence in everything: products, strategies, systems, processes and people (Bounds *et al.* 1994)	*Differences in quality amount to differences in the quantity of some desired ingredient or attribute* (Abbott 1955)			
Manufacturing	Fine craftsmanship and a rejection of mass production (Lewis 1984)	The list of specifications to which the product as well as ingredients and components have to conform (Van Gigch 1977)	*Conformance to specifications* (Levitt 1972) *The degree to which a specific product conforms to a design or specification* (Gilmore 1974)		
Consumer	Quality is the goodness or excellence of some thing. It is assessed against accepted standards of merit	The totality of features and characteristics of a product or service that bear on its ability to satisfy stated or implied needs	The consistent conformance to customer expectations (Lew Lehr quoted in Anderson 1988)	*Fitness for use* (Juran 1988) *Meeting the customer requirements* (Oakland 2000)	

	for such things and against the interests/needs of users and other stakeholders (Smith 1993)	(International Standards Organisation – see Freund 1985)	Quality can be defined as conformance to specifications for output that is tangible and standardized. For output that is customized and intangible, quality can be defined as the extent to which the output meets and/or exceeds customer expectations (Reeves and Bednar 1994)	*Delighting the customer* (Peters and Austin 1985) *Meeting or exceeding customer expectations* (Gronroos 1983)	*Affordable excellence* *The presence of value defined by the customer* (Federal Express)
Value	Quality is the degree of excellence at an acceptable price and the control of variability at an acceptable cost (Broh 1982)	The amounts of the unpriced attributes contained in each unit of the priced attribute (Leffler 1982)	A predictable degree of uniformity and dependability at a low cost suited to the market (Deming 1986) Minimizing the loss imparted to the society from the time a product is shipped (Taguchi 1986)	The degree of conformance of all the relevant features and characteristics of the product (or service) to all aspects of a customer's need, limited by the price and delivery he or she will accept (Groocock 1986)	

industry. Such definitions give clear guidance to employees on what is required and lend themselves particularly well to statistical process control. It is also relatively easy to check whether the specifications have in fact been achieved. The main problem with manufacturing definitions is that there is no guarantee that the specifications set are what customers actually want. As Berry *et al.* (1988) point out, 'quality is conformance to customer specifications; it is the customer's definition of quality, not management's, that counts'. An example of this is a branch of McDonald's the author worked with a few years ago. By coincidence this store was visited on the very same day by senior staff from the region (incognito) and by an independent mystery shopper employed by the company. Senior staff rated it very highly – 'one of the best in the region' – whereas the mystery shopper looking at the same service from the customer's view saw many shortcomings. Clearly the outlet met the company's specifications, but not the customer's.

Examples in the public sector include housing managers who see themselves as the expert, rather than in partnership with the resident, and a clinician who defines quality without reference to the patient's experience and wishes.

Consumer-based

Consumer-based ('user-based' is Garvin's original term) approaches aim to avoid the internal focus which often arises with a manufacturing-based definition. Juran's (1988) and Oakland's (2000) definitions given in Table 1.2 make it clear that it is the customer's concept of quality that matters. These definitions have been extended in a number of different ways. Tom Peters says that satisfying customers is not enough: 'We don't want to satisfy the customer, we want to thrill the customer, we want to delight the customer!' (Peters and Austin 1985) while Judd and Winder (1995) add that quality also involves 'being responsive to their full range of needs and assisting in the fulfilment of those needs'.

Gronroos (1983) takes note of the importance of customer expectations in their perception of quality, while there is much evidence (e.g. Haywood-Farmer 1988) that customers judge quality by comparing their perceptions of a service to their expectations of what the service should be like. Another reason for including expectations is that 'when quality is simply a matter of meeting specifications or requirements, it becomes static. If we treat quality as a matter of meeting expectations, then it forces management to seek continuous improvement' (Foggin 1991).

However, consumer-based definitions do not explicitly take account of the price that customers have to pay for their goods and services. This has led some authors to define quality using the value-based approach.

Value-based

The essence of the value-based approach can be seen from the following statement by Feigenbaum (1991): 'Quality does not have the popular meaning of "best" in any abstract sense . . . It is that quality which establishes the proper balance between the cost of the product or service and the customer value it renders'. This approach makes the relationship between cost and quality explicit and will be of much more help to organizations in non-premium markets than the transcendent and product approaches. There is a danger however in such definitions that a company uses its low price as an excuse for not providing what the customer requires. For example, goods with a 5 per cent defect rate, or a flight or train journey with long delays, even if offered at very low prices, might offer value to a particular customer but since they do not meet the customer's requirements they cannot be seen as quality products or services.

Hybrid definitions

As the above discussion indicates, while each of these approaches has its merits, none encapsulates all aspects of quality that need to be included. Many authors have instead used definitions which are essentially hybrids in the sense that they take some aspects from two or more of the above definitions.

Examples of such 'hybrid' definitions are given in Table 1.2. As an example of how to interpret the table, the definition by Broh is a hybrid of the value and transcendent approaches. The very fact that there are hybrids for each combination confirms the variety of and lack of consensus on the definitions that have been recommended.

Defining quality in health and social care

While most of the above discussion is very relevant to the public and voluntary sectors, the definitions were developed primarily for organizations in the private sector. To see their relevance to health and social care, this section first examines four such definitions from the management literature:

- *Fitness for purpose* (Juran 1986 – consumer-based). This definition can be very useful when considering which drugs or equipment to use. If an item fits the purpose for which it is intended then it is a quality product. On the other hand, if an item embodies the latest technology but is not suitable for the task in hand then, in this context, it is of poor quality. In maternity services for example, for a woman who wishes to be free to move around in labour, the most sophisticated monitoring equipment, with all its trailing wires, will be less appropriate than a simple sonic aid. While the aid will provide less information to clinicians, it is arguably a better quality service for the mother, since it will allow her to do as she wishes. Overall, though, this definition clearly has its roots in manufacturing and does not transfer over very well to the service sector.

- *Conformance to specifications* (Levitt 1972 – manufacturing-based). Conformance to specifications or standards sounds commendable, but it does beg the question of who sets the specifications in the first place. If they reflect both the views of professionals and the needs and expectations of service users, then they may be fine. In practice, where such definitions are used, this is generally not the case.
- *Conformance to requirements* (Crosby 1984 – consumer-based). Crosby's definition seems fine but it does not say anything about costs. Patients in hospital may, for example, want their own room complete with private telephone, satellite television and space for all the family; housing tenants may want the latest Jacuzzi; many social service users may want support every hour of every day. Where these people do not pay directly for the service, the organization has to balance the needs of individuals with those of other potential users, given the funding available to it. Donabedian (1980) concludes: 'I believe that in real life we do not have the option of excluding monetary costs from the individualised definition of quality'.
- *Meeting customer requirements and expectations at an acceptable price* (Moullin 1995 – consumer/value hybrid). This definition, unlike the others, does consider the relationship between meeting customers' requirements and cost, an issue very relevant for health and social care. It also makes explicit the importance of customer expectations. However, the use of the term 'price', and perhaps also the word 'customer', may be somewhat problematical since the customers who benefit may not be the same as those who pay.

None of the above definitions perfectly match the circumstances of health and social care. The following definition of quality in the public sector is from Øvretveit (1990) although in fact his definition adds the words 'and purchasers' at the end: 'Fully meeting the needs of those who need the service most, at the lowest cost to the organisation, within limits and directives set by higher authorities'. Most people working in public services in particular would I feel give a sigh of relief that the phrase 'within the limits and directives' has been included. Public sector organizations do have responsibilities placed upon them that are essentially non-negotiable and have to work within these. For example, in social care, work with children and families is carried out in the context of the Children Act 1989 and it is frequently not possible to meet the wishes of a parent where these are incompatible with the needs of the child. It is important to recognize that this definition can only be valid if those 'higher authorities' genuinely have the commitment to put the needs of patients, service users, carers and staff at the forefront.

Another key phrase here is 'those who need the service most'. The idea behind this is that there may not be sufficient resources to meet everyone's needs – for example, in housing and health. One could argue, with justification, that more resources should be provided, but there will be a point where there are insufficient resources to meet everyone's needs.

The definition of quality recommended in this book for the public and voluntary sectors is as follows: 'Meeting the requirements and expectations of service users and other stakeholders while keeping costs to a minimum'. An alternative definition, which might suit some health services, would be 'meeting the requirements and expectations of patients, carers and other stakeholders while keeping costs to a minimum'.

Quality in primary care

The use of this definition is illustrated by the following example of what quality would mean in a general practitioner (GP) surgery. McSweeney (1997), following on from some earlier work by Toon (1994), gives four possible models of quality for primary care: the biomedical model, the teleological model, the preventive model and the business model – see Table 1.3.

Which model corresponds most closely to 'meeting the requirements and expectations of service users and other stakeholders'? Clearly no surgery could function without the biomedical approach, but what about the others? Some people will have strong views that a particular model must be adopted. However, with the above definition of quality, there is no ambiguity. Given that most patients wish to have their symptoms relieved, to be treated with empathy and compassion, to be offered screening or other preventive services, *and* to have acceptable waiting times, the GP surgery needs to address *all* of these issues simultaneously. So all four models are relevant – and that is the extent of the challenge of managing quality in health and public services.

Table 1.3 Models of quality in primary care

Model	Definition
Biomedical	Correction of biological dysfunction through accurate clinical diagnosis. Appropriate relief of symptoms and cure from disease.
Teleological	Viewing the patient from a more holistic perspective, helping them understand their illness. Being empathetic and compassionate. Offering privacy, dignity and confidentiality.
Preventive	Offering services which prevent disease or lower risk (e.g. immunization and screening). Promoting healthier lifestyles.
Business	Offering an expanding menu of services (e.g. counselling, physiotherapy, blood tests) on the premises. Convenient appointments and acceptable waiting times. Attractive decor. Well-designed layout.

Source: McSweeny (1997).

Dimensions of quality: identifying the needs of service users and other stakeholders

Given that quality is meeting the needs of service users, it is not enough to satisfy some requirements but not others. In banking, for example, it is not sufficient to offer a good range of services if many people want to use the bank at weekends or after work and it is closed at those times. Similarly, excellent medical treatment in a hospital may not lead to patient satisfaction if people have had to wait an unreasonable time before being admitted, if they have arrived anxious due to lack of car parking, or if they did not receive any explanation of what was going to happen to them. As Jan Carlzon (1987), the chief executive of Scandinavian Airlines put it, 'Excellent service is about being 1 per cent better at 100 things not 100 per cent better at one thing'.

As an example, consider what would influence airline passengers in a decision about whether or not to travel with a particular airline on a subsequent occasion. A wide variety of factors might affect this decision, including safety, flight timing (convenience and no delays), price, ease of transport to airport, car parking, check-in, passport control, shops and café facilities at the airport, friendliness of cabin crew, baggage handling and quality of in-flight food and entertainment. Moreover if they had a disability, there would be an additional set of needs that would have to be met. Overall, from the airline's point of view, there is no shortage of opportunities to disappoint their customers.

However, despite all the different factors an airline has to deal with, its task is very straightforward compared with that of service providers in public services. While an airline does have to make some trade-offs between the needs of business and holiday clients, it does not have anything like the wide range of customers and stakeholders with different and often conflicting requirements. The following situation, based on Casson and Manning (1997: 58–9), illustrates this complexity:

> A teacher noticed that a 9-year-old boy had bruising on the back of his legs and contacted a social worker. When asked what had happened, the boy said that the bruising was caused by his mother's live-in partner when he had misbehaved. The child lives in overcrowded accommodation with his five siblings. His mother's partner is not his father, but he is the father of the two youngest children. Whose needs and views does the social worker have to take into account in assessing this situation and what are their requirements?

Table 1.4 shows the service users and other stakeholders involved in this situation, each with different requirements that need to be taken into account. While a good social worker may end up satisfying all the clients and stakeholders in this situation, there are many cases where this will not be

Table 1.4   Requirements of service users and stakeholders

Service user/stakeholder	What they want
The child	To feel safe at home Not to be hit His mother to protect him from being hit
The mother/carer	For her partner to love her and care for her and her children For her children to be safe and secure Decent housing and enough money to live on
The mother's partner	For the children to obey him and their mother To love and care for the mother and children Decent housing and enough money to live on
The teacher	Reassurance that the child is being properly cared for so he can learn and her class will do well
Senior social services managers in the department	To be assured that the department is doing its job properly and that resources are being used effectively
The community	Assurance that children in need will be helped and kept safe Assurance that everyone will be treated equitably
The Department of Health	Adherence to legislation and guidance
The social worker	To prevent the child being assaulted again while keeping him at home and in his community To provide effective support to the family so that the children can develop to their full potential

possible. In child protection it is particularly important that the child's needs are not ignored, as the other clients and stakeholders have more power than the child. This is very different from the airline situation.

While a simple brainstorming exercise would enable a team to identify most aspects of quality relevant to its service users, it is also likely to leave some out. A framework, such as that given by Berry *et al.* (1988), can be of assistance here. The authors conducted extensive in-depth interviews with a wide variety of customer groups in the service sector to find out what is important to them. Classifying the results, they found that customers assessed quality in terms of a number of factors, or 'dimensions of quality'. These are listed in the left-hand column of Table 1.5, with good and bad examples of each factor in the two other columns.

The ten dimensions of quality shown in Table 1.5 vary in terms of how easy or difficult it is to evaluate them. For example, a dental patient can

Table 1.5 Dimensions of service quality

Factor	Good examples	Bad examples
Reliability	IT services always available at the required times.	Failure to phone service user back as agreed.
Responsiveness	Maintenance staff who service equipment at short notice.	Long queues.
Competence	Staff carry out task with skill.	Staff inadequately trained for the task in hand.
Access	Easy to find one's way, easy to get to. Accessible to people with disabilities.	Poor signing. Limited car parking.
Courtesy	Polite and helpful staff.	Senior staff patronizing and condescending.
Communication	Medical staff who explain diagnosis and alternative treatments without jargon.	Lack of information about what is happening or what is likely to happen.
Credibility	Staff you feel you can trust and depend on.	Staff who you feel have not been given the correct information.
Security	A feeling of personal safety and confidentiality.	Unlit access at night.
Understanding/ knowing the customer	Staff who make an effort to meet a patient's individual requirements.	Staff who don't recognize a regular service user.
Tangibles	Pleasing physical appearance of facilities.	Poor or out-of-date equipment being used for the service.

Source: Berry *et al.* (1988).

evaluate the tangibles – a filling or gold tooth – fairly easily and also whether or not the staff were friendly. However, issues such as competence are difficult, if not impossible, to evaluate. While the list of dimensions of quality is very applicable to public services, organizations in the public sector have additional values that are central to their beliefs and should therefore be included. As Pfeffer and Coote (1991) point out, these include equity and equality, empowerment, involvement of staff and public participation.

Maxwell (1984) identified six dimensions of quality which could apply to both health and social care: equity, access to services, relevance to need, efficiency, social acceptability and effectiveness. For health services, these have been superseded by the NHS Performance Assessment Framework (NHS Executive 1999b) which aims to encapsulate what health services need to provide for users and other stakeholders (see Table 1.6). Note that both Maxwell's dimensions and the Framework differ from Berry's list in that they are intended to reflect the needs of all stakeholders, not just patients and service users.

Table 1.6 The NHS Performance Assessment Framework

Area	Aspects of performance
Health improvement	The overall health of populations, reflecting social and environmental factors and individual behaviour as well as care provided by the NHS and other agencies.
Fair access	The fairness of the provision of services in relation to need on various dimensions: geographical, socioeconomic, demographic (age, ethnicity, sex) and care groups (e.g. people with learning difficulties).
Effective delivery of appropriate health care	The extent to which services are clinically effective, appropriate to need, timely, in line with agreed standards, provided according to best practice and delivered by appropriately trained and educated staff.
Efficiency	The extent to which the NHS provides efficient services, including: cost per unit of care/outcome, productivity of capital estate and labour productivity.
Patient/carer experience	The patient/carer perceptions on the delivery of services including responsiveness to individual needs and preferences; the skill, care and continuity of service provision; patient involvement, good information and choice; waiting times and accessibility; the physical environment; the organization and courtesy of administrative arrangements.
Health outcomes of NHS care	NHS success in using its resources to reduce levels of risk factors, disease, impairment and complications of treatment; improve quality of life for patients and carers; and reduce premature deaths.

Source: NHS Executive (1999b).

While the effective delivery of appropriate health care will be uppermost in most patients' minds, it is important not to underestimate the importance of the patient and carer experience. For example, Harr (2001) cites research evidence from Switzerland which revealed that only 15 per cent of patients who changed their dentist did so due to poor quality of work or high cost. In contrast, 70 per cent gave the reason as poor service or lack of courtesy among the practice staff. Harr, whose dental practice was a prize-winner of the European Quality Award in 2000, infers that the quality of the treatment provided is taken for granted by patients and that attention is needed to friendliness of staff, reducing waiting times, providing information and re-assurance, creating a congenial atmosphere and other service aspects. Trent Regional Health Authority's work on what they have called a 'patient centreometer' aims to unpick this dimension of the Performance Assessment Framework. They worked closely with users and carers to identify the factors that are indicative of a 'patient-centred NHS', which they classified under the following headings:

- patients in control of their care;
- services integrated across agencies and professions;
- services that do the 'small things that matter' well;
- services that are sensitive, equal, fair and listen and act.

A key aspect of putting patients in control of their care is the provision of information, both about their illness and about alternative forms of treatment. Many health professionals prefer not to mention risks associated with treatments or alternative forms of treatment, with the aim of not upsetting patients or making them anxious. However, Joanne Rule, chief executive of Cancer Bacup, says, 'What doctors need to understand is that though choice can be upsetting, it is also empowering and helps to restore the self-esteem that takes such a battering in someone with a serious illness' (Feinnman 2001). Feinnman agrees, saying that 'recent research shows that nearly nine out of 10 people want as much information as possible from their doctor, good or bad, so that they can participate in planning their own health care'. However, it is also important not to ignore the one in ten patients who may prefer the traditional method and a sensitive approach is needed.

Involving users and carers is very important in establishing user require-ments and expectations. It is often tempting to feel that as 'experts' staff know what their service users want. However, talking to service users directly and getting them to describe what they want in their own words will almost always provide fresh insights. This is illustrated by the outcomes of a work-shop carried out in Sheffield with people with learning difficulties. This workshop identified the following characteristics that people with learning difficulties want from their support workers:

- Not giving us the message that we are 'mental'.
- They should be trained in communication skills and have the time to listen and talk.
- We don't want staff who don't want to listen or who pretend to listen. We want staff who listen and talk to us in a way we understand.
- The right support worker would use plain language and no jargon. They should use audiotapes, large print, sign language, makaton, Braille and other means of saying things when they need to.
- The right support worker would respect our relationships and keep what we say private.
- The right support worker should be a person who is there – someone to turn to.

- It would be useful to have pictures and symbols that stand for words. Everyone should use the same pictures.
- Not to tell us what to do in our lives.
- Not control what we do in our lives (e.g. you *have* to go to a day centre).
- We can tell you what we want. Sometimes we need to know a lot of things to choose for ourselves.
- Enough money for good, well-trained, well-paid staff. We can help with training.
- The right for people with learning difficulties to buy in help that is right for them.
- We want to help choose, interview and select the people who work with us.

In home care, a study by the Joseph Rowntree Foundation (2000) involving users gave the following characteristics of a quality home-care service: staff reliability; continuity of care and of staff; kindness and understanding of care workers; cheerfulness and demeanour of care staff; competence in undertaking specific tasks; flexibility to respond to changing needs and requirements; and knowledge and experience of the needs and wishes of the service user. Another study, carried out by the National Institute for Social Work (2000) identified what service users and carers value from social work:

> People using services value workers who: recognise and build on people's own expertise and experience, their culture, history and religion; treat people equally and with respect, are open and honest even when the news is bad, provide information to enable people to make choices and stay in as much control over their lives as possible; develop more equal relationships between workers and users and enable people to work out what they want to do.

Quality for users of an artificial limb centre

For amputees using an artificial limb centre, there are five key dimensions of service quality:

- *Comfort*: comfortable, good fit, ease of use, lightweight.
- *Function*: usefulness, range of motion, durability, health of residual limb after using the prosthesis, ability to resume desired activities, psychosocial well-being, energy required in using the prosthesis.
- *Appearance*: pleasing to look at, status and respect of one's peers, visual and auditory considerations.
- *Service*: right first time, reasonable waiting time, appropriate follow-up, complaint resolution.
- *Communication*: involvement in process, information given.

According to Kwong (2001), 'it may be controversial to put communication as one of the quality attributes; however I believe that this can affect the amputees' perception on the quality of prosthesis'. This is backed up by Kalter *et al.* (1989) who say that the quality of life an amputee is able to maintain is in part related to the prosthesis quality, which results from proper fitting, regular adjustment and the utilization of new technologies. However, it is also necessary for the prosthetist to be aware of the concerns of the amputee and the ways in which prosthetic services can address these concerns most effectively. Indeed, a later research study by Neilsen (1991) showed that amputees wish to plan treatment in partnership with the prosthetist and to have more information provided. Specifically, amputees wanted highly qualified technical care from a professional who communicates a real interest in their needs.

In contrast to these findings, a questionnaire carried out on all staff in the Artificial Limb Centre at Tan Tock Seng Hospital in Singapore showed that only 15 per cent of staff agreed that communication with the amputee was important to the amputee's perception of the quality of the prosthesis; 25 per cent were neutral, while 50 per cent disagreed and 10 per cent strongly disagreed (Kwong 2001). This appears to indicate a wide gap in their understanding of user expectations.

Dimensions of quality for carers

To deliver a quality service, organizations in health and social care need to meet not only the needs of patients and service users, but also those of carers. Carers' needs include the following (Department of Health 1999c):

- well-being of the person being cared for;
- freedom to have a life of their own;
- maintaining their own health;
- confidence in services;
- a say in service provision.

A recent publication from the National Schizophrenia Fellowship (2001), *Commitment to Carers*, identifies four different dimensions of quality for carers of people with mental health problems. While they were developed for carers of mental health users, the four headings (recognition and understanding, support, information and involvement) could apply to all types of carer. Details of what relatives, partners and friends should expect from mental health services under each of these dimensions, as outlined in *Commitment to Carers*, are given in Table 1.7.

What customers want

To finish this section, the following list of what customers want comes from Nissan UK (David 1988), but is probably even more relevant to health and social care than to manufacturing industry.

Table 1.7 Dimensions of quality for carers of people with mental health needs

Recognition and understanding	You should be recognized and listened to as a partner in providing care.
	You should be valued as someone dedicated to helping the person you care for and who knows them well.
	You should be treated with courtesy and respected for your skills (e.g. overseeing their medication).
	You should be able to work with staff who understand the effects of mental illness on yourself and your family.
	You should be able to request an appointment with the consultant psychiatrist or another mental health professional.
Support	You should receive help and information when it first becomes evident that you are providing care for someone with a mental health problem.
	You should have the chance to discuss your concerns about the person's illness and how it is affecting you.
	You should receive prompt and positive responses to your requests for help.
	You should be able to get immediate help in a crisis.
	You should have your needs assessed as well as those of the person you care for and have them reviewed periodically.
	You should be able to have breaks from caring.
	You should be given access to help in communicating with staff (e.g. interpreter, signer).
Information	You should be given an explanation of the mental health problem affecting the person you care for and be told where you can go to get more information.
	You should be told what treatments the person is receiving, what other treatments are available, how they work and what the potential side-effects are.
	You should be told what services are available for the person you care for, such as day care and employment services.
	You should be told how to recognize signs of a relapse.
	You should be told who to contact in an emergency and be given a 24-hour phone number.
	You should be given advice on how you can best cope with the effects of the mental health problem at critical times such as home leave and the period following discharge.
	You should be given information about what support will be provided when you are no longer able to provide care yourself.
Involvement	You should expect that mental health staff will encourage the person to allow their carer to be involved unless that person has clearly expressed the wish to exclude you.
	You should be able to give your views and have your questions answered about the care plan.
	You should be able to have someone with you at meetings to help you put your views across.
	You should have the opportunity to be involved in the planning and development of services in your area.
	You should be able to choose whether you are prepared to accept the role of carer.

Source: National Schizophrenia Fellowship (2001).

- Don't ignore me
- Make me feel wanted
- Don't lie to me
- Give me clear information
- Don't insult my intelligence
- Keep your promises
- Don't keep me waiting
- Listen to me when I tell you how to improve your services
- Be sensitive to my needs
- Treat me fairly – don't rip me off

Perceptions and expectations

The definition of quality used in this book refers to the 'requirements and expectations of service users'. There are a number of reasons for including 'expectations' in the definition. First, this gives a dynamic element to the definition, because as expectations change user satisfaction with the same service may well change. Second, it makes clear the importance of expectations on the perceptions of service users. This can be seen from the following three pointers from Parasuraman *et al.* (1985) which are based on in-depth interviews with a wide range of customer groups.

- *Consumers' perceptions of service quality result from a comparison of their expectations before they receive service with their actual experience of the service.* The quality of a service or product is not just determined by the customer's reaction to it – it also depends on the customer's expectations. A patient who has not been told that a particular procedure would be painful, or a woman who expected a social worker to get her a benefit she is not entitled to, would both feel that they had not received a quality service. Taking time to explain to the patient what is likely to happen to them or informing the woman about the role of the social worker, while not actually affecting the outcomes in each case, would have a significant positive impact on the user's perceptions of the quality of the service: 'Customers judge quality by comparing their perceptions of what they receive to their expectations of what they should receive. This is important in understanding and controlling service quality. A customer who waits knowing it will be 30 minutes before s/he is served, may be happier than one who waits half as long but does not know how long that wait will be' (Haywood-Farmer 1988).
- *Quality perceptions are derived from the service process as well as from the service outcome.* This is, of course, well recognized by staff in both health and social care. For example, while returning home from the maternity unit with a healthy, bouncing baby is naturally of prime importance to new parents, it is certainly not the only quality criterion for them. What kind of a time they had and how they were treated will be remembered for

the rest of their lives. Similarly, in a residential home for children with learning difficulties, it is not just educational progress and development that is important but also how the children are cared for.

- *Service quality is of two types: normal and exceptional.* First, there is the level of quality at which the normal service is delivered (e.g. services for 'standard' patients). Second, there is the quality level at which 'exceptions' or 'problems' are handled. If something goes wrong for a patient or service user, whether or not the organization is at fault, how well is this dealt with? Also, how easy is it for them to complain and how is that complaint dealt with? Another aspect of this is the experience of patients and service users with disabilities or non-standard needs. Do they just have to fit in with the system or are their individual needs met? These factors are also important to quality of service.

Moments of truth

The term 'moments of truth' was popularized by Jan Carlzon, who was chief executive of Scandinavian Airlines. He recognized that the customer's perception of an airline was based on a combination of the many interactions and services received: getting a convenient flight, arriving at the airport, parking the car, queueing at the check-in gate, waiting in the airport lounge, the food received, the attention of the cabin staff, safety and timing of the flight and retrieving luggage at the end of the flight:

> Last year, each of our 10 million customers came into contact with approximately 5 SAS employees and this contact lasted an average of 15 seconds each time. Thus SAS is 'created' in the minds of our customers 50 million times a year, 15 seconds at a time. These 50 million 'moments of truth' are the moments that ultimately determine whether SAS will succeed or fail as a company. They are moments when we must prove to our customers that SAS is their best alternative.
>
> (Carlzon 1987)

The term 'moment of truth' is a bullfighting metaphor coined by Normann *et al.* (1978). Perceived quality is realized at the moment of truth, when the service provider and the service customer confront one another in the arena. At every moment of truth there are three possible outcomes:

- the customer will get less than they expect and be disappointed or angry;
- the customer will get exactly what they expect and therefore not be dissatisfied;
- the customer gets service of a higher quality than they expect and are delighted.

In a large service organization like a hospital there will be tens of thousands of moments of truth every day. In most cases the employees involved may be low level and not particularly well paid. But it is their performance and the support they receive from elsewhere in the organization which will determine how that organization will be perceived by its customers.

This concept is probably even more relevant to many parts of the public sector than to an airline. Service users will typically encounter a range of staff from different departments and agencies. While customers of an airline may well be anxious about flying, this is not comparable to the vulnerability many patients and service users feel. The words of a doctor or a kind volunteer in a drop-in centre may be remembered for a very long time.

There will be a large number of moments of truth that will influence service users' perceptions of the service. Organizations in the public and private sectors alike need to manage all these moments of truth to ensure they give customers or users a positive experience.

Quality and equity

Equity and quality go hand in hand. It may be some consolation for people to know that everyone else is getting the same poor service, but true equity is about making sure that all groups of people, regardless of ethnic origin, social class, gender or sexual orientation, receive services which meet their needs and sensitively take into account their circumstances and the particular pressures upon them.

Equity is one of the core values of the NHS, social services departments and most voluntary organizations in the care sector: 'Without [quality] there is unfairness. Every patient who is treated in the NHS wants to know that they can rely on receiving high quality care when they need it' (Department of Health 1997). To achieve equity, staff have to be proactive, as discrimination can be subtle. For example, the complaints policy of a hospital may appear to be quite well-run and patients who complain might be fairly satisfied with the response. However, if on analysing these complaints it becomes clear that there are many more complaints from articulate white middle-class families than from other groups, the service needs to evaluate how it can get similar feedback from those other groups and thereby be able to respond to their wishes too.

Another example is a social worker working with the single mother of a teenager in trouble with the police. The mother is of African Caribbean origin and wishes her son to be placed in local authority care. In order to treat the family equitably, the worker will need to take into account the issues surrounding ethnicity and other circumstances of the family – and in particular to be alert to possibilities of racism. The social worker would also need to be aware of their own attitudes to race and racism. In mental health, the following guideline from the UK mental health charity MIND is very useful:

A mental health service should be equally accessible and available to everyone in the community that it serves . . . mental health services must not discriminate against people on the grounds that they are old . . . nor that they are from certain ethnic groups . . . nor that they are gay . . . nor on any other irrelevant grounds.

(Harding and Beresford 1996)

Accessibility is a very important part of equity. It does not just refer to appropriate access for disabled people, car parking and clear signing in a hospital – although, of course, these are important too. The forms required to apply for services, for example, are also part of the accessibility of the service and are often unnecessarily intimidating. One organization, for instance, sent pensioners a 16-page form to apply for a disabled facilities grant towards the cost of a chairlift for stairs.

Another aspect of equity is to make sure that different groups within the community a department or area of activity is intended to serve do, in fact, make use of the service. It is important to find out whether some groups make less use of the service, relative to their needs, than others. For example, in Sheffield, it was found that in the Manor area near the centre of the city, three times as many people experienced chest pain symptoms compared with the more affluent suburb of Dore. However, the number of people receiving certain types of treatment for heart disease was twice as high in Dore as in the Manor. Low take-up of a service among some groups may be because they do not know the service exists or because they do not feel it is for them. In order to make a service truly equitable, staff need to find ways of changing this pattern, preferably through consultation with the particular group that is under-represented.

Equity is also about providing culturally appropriate services. In residential homes or meals-on-wheels services, for example, roast beef is an excellent choice for many people, but it may be seen by some Hindus as showing a marked lack of respect for their culture. The language barrier can also be extremely frustrating. The chief executive of one hospital trust wrote to staff saying that, as the interpreting service for certain languages cost £17 per hour, it had to be used 'very sparingly'. How consultants could be expected to prescribe the right treatment for patients who are unable to explain their symptoms was not made clear! In social care, too, where communication is all-important, overcoming the language barrier is vital. Having to rely on family members to interpret, which is not uncommon, is generally a breach of confidentiality and particularly inappropriate if that family member is a child. The Newham Black and Ethnic Minority Community Care Forum has a useful comment to make on this issue:

> For black and ethnic minority users and carers, a language barrier hinders a prompt and effective service. People are sent to different sections without understanding why; procedures are not explained to them so that they can understand; they do not get the interpreting help they need and have to rely on a relative or child, which is quite unacceptable and lacks confidentiality.

(Harding and Beresford 1996)

Quality and cost

The relationship between quality and cost is often misunderstood. The following comments are perhaps typical: 'We can't afford to improve quality, we're already likely to be over budget as it is'; 'How can we afford to improve quality when we can't even afford a decent . . .'. However, the relationship between quality and cost is not so clear-cut. Most improvements in quality will cost money, but many can be seen as an investment which will repay itself many times over in a short space of time.

It is not difficult to think of examples where improving quality costs more. Upgrading existing facilities or extending the opening hours of a drop-in clinic will both carry a price tag. However, other costs may be reduced. For example, better X-ray or ultrasound imaging equipment may lead to more people being diagnosed correctly or sooner, reducing the cost of patient stays in hospital. Similarly, better facilities for staff may reduce absenteeism and turnover, saving recruitment and training costs.

Reducing medical errors or the proportion of X-ray retakes are clear examples of improved quality leading to reduced costs. In social care too, giving more support to a family could avoid the high costs associated with family breakdown. As the Department of Health's *Working Together to Safeguard Children* document (1999b) says, 'Providing services and support to children and families under stress may strengthen the capacity of parents to respond to the needs of their children before problems develop into abuse'.

In many cases, the service needs to be viewed as a whole, because a given improvement in quality may incur additional costs for one budget holder, while the reduction in costs will manifest itself in a different department's budget.

The prevention, appraisal, failure (PAF) model

The PAF model identifies four main cost elements associated with quality:

- *Costs of prevention*: these are the costs associated with preventing poor quality before it happens and include more attention to product and service design, employee training and developing a proper quality management programme. They include the costs of training on quality, time spent in quality improvement meetings, writing procedures and specifications for quality and better facilities.
- *Costs of appraisal*: these include the costs of checking that items received conform to requirements, checking the processes involved in delivering the service, and confirming the quality of the completed work. Instead it would be better if quality was built into the process and controlled by those directly involved. An example is the time spent chasing staff in another department to make sure it has done what it is supposed to have done. In most cases it would be cheaper if that department kept people

regularly informed about progress rather than expecting them to do the chasing.

- *Internal failure costs*: these comprise the resources involved in rectifying a service which was performed incorrectly, but does not directly affect the main outcome for the service user. An example would be where relevant information was not available at a case conference, leading to wasted staff time, or incorrect specifications for pathology tests which have to be returned to the issuing clinical staff for clarification. No one enjoys having their mistakes pointed out, so people should be encouraged to get it right first time, through better training, processes, equipment and support.
- *External failure costs*: these are the costs of mistakes discovered by patients and service users or which directly affect them. They often cannot be put right after the event and can lead to devastating effects on the people concerned. It is difficult to quantify the costs of poor quality in health and social care because they are human costs, often paid for by patients, service users or carers as a reduction in their quality of life or potential.

Two further costs of external failure are those of dealing with customer complaints and litigation. In 1998/9 for example there were 124,000 written complaints about family health services or hospital care in the UK, while the NHS paid out around £400 million in clinical litigation settlements. In addition, in more serious cases, failure can result in the loss of confidence and goodwill, damaging the corporate image of the organization. The poor quality of certain heart operations at Bristol Royal Infirmary in the 1990s, and the inadequacy of the hospital's quality processes which should have identified and dealt with the problem much earlier, caused considerable damage to the reputation of the hospital.

The PAF model shows that a quality improvement programme will increase prevention costs, but may also lead to reductions in other cost elements, as shown in Figure 1.1. The Department of Trade and Industry (1990) concluded that 'Evidence suggests that quality-related costs may be reduced to one-third of their present level, within a period of three years, by the commitment of the organisation to a process of continuous quality'. This is the basis for the often-quoted statement by Philip Crosby – one of the quality gurus – that 'quality is free' (Crosby 1984). In fact it would be more correct to say that quality is an investment with an immediate pay-off.

To take a very simple example, one local authority social work team of six people, four full-time and two part-time, shared two telephones between them. This resulted in the following costs of failure: delays due to people not being able to use the phone to arrange visits and delays in people trying to contact the team. All in all there was a lot of wasted time. The costs of prevention would have been just that of additional phones.

At the other end of the scale, the Department of Health (2000a) estimates that adverse events in which harm is caused to patients cost the service an estimated £2 billion a year in additional hospital stays alone, without taking

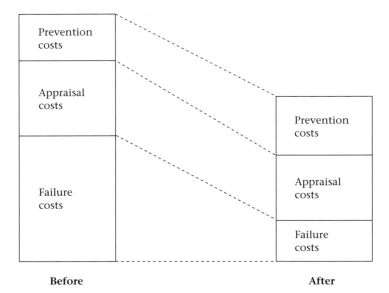

Before   **After**

Figure 1.1   Costs of quality before and after quality improvement

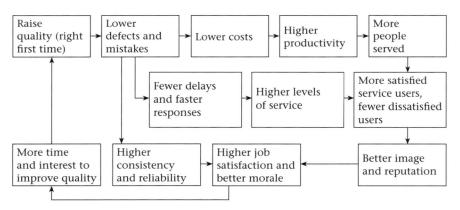

Figure 1.2   The effect of improving quality
Source: Øvretveit (1990).

any account of human or wider economic costs. As Goasdoue (1990) puts it, 'If you are serious about quality, you have to understand that preventing problems is a low but unavoidable expense, and fixing them after they have happened is high and avoidable'.

Figure 1.2, adapted from Øvretveit (1990), shows the effect of improving quality.

There has been much attention to the costs of poor quality in the NHS. Hugh Koch (1991) summarizes the issue for health service managers very well: 'Failure costs are unproductive, unnecessary and make the service less attractive, uncompetitive and unacceptable to patients, relatives and referring agencies. The effort to make services right first time is less costly than carrying out a process, e.g. taking an X-ray, postcoding, blood test, two or three times'.

The following case study, based on Iles (1990), illustrates the benefits of tackling a recurrent problem in any organization.

Missing reports in outpatients

St Andrew's Hospital in Newham in the East End of London had a major problem with missing pathology and other reports in the outpatient department. Surveys indicated that in some clinics between 20 and 25 per cent of results were missing when required. This was causing much wasted time and resentment from nurses, doctors and pathology staff, not to mention the patients.

On examining what was going wrong it was found that the pathology clerk 'could not tell which results were required or whether any results were missing. Missing results were identified as such only during the clinic session after the patient had arrived and often while the patient was already in consultation with the doctor' (Iles 1990).

To tackle this problem the outpatients manager worked closely with all staff involved, including doctors, to produce a plan which documented clearly the roles of all involved. This centred on a new form for future appointment requirements. As the patient attends the clinic, the doctor ticks the reports required at the next visit. When a particular report is available a tick is inserted in red next to that inserted by the doctor, so that missing reports can be clearly identified.

The costs of this initiative were not negligible. The time spent by the outpatient manager, the doctors and others involved cost money. These are the costs of prevention. Costs saved included the costs of appraisal – in particular, nursing time spent enquiring whether results were ready. This had previously been so extensive that an agency nurse was required on busy clinic days to offset the time wasted. This had cost £3120 per annum. Also saved were the costs of internal failure. These included time wasted by the doctors often having to interrupt or postpone their consultations because they could not decide on the appropriate treatment for the patient, and also time wasted by pathology staff. In addition there was the disruption and the effect on the morale of all staff involved. The external costs saved included the fact that patients no longer had to wait until their results were found. Also, patients had previously needed to make another appointment if results were not available, so even more time and energy was wasted. In addition, patients now see the outpatient clinic as an 'organized and efficient establishment which enhances their confidence in us and their satisfaction with their treatment' (Iles 1990). Overall then, the savings made by this quality improvement programme are many times that of the costs of prevention. In this case quality really does save money!

Bridging the quality gap

Service quality is a dynamic factor: the expectations of patients and service users are continually rising and the service package needs to keep up with them. Just as a personal computer with the power and speed that people found satisfactory five years ago would today be seen as offering poor quality, so the level of service provided five years ago will not be sufficient now. An organization should continually anticipate the needs of service users and patients and provide them with 'that little bit extra' – a reduction in waiting time, clearer information about what is likely to happen, a warmer welcome.

Although many service organizations are improving the quality of the service they provide, it may not be perceived to be any better than it was. Indeed, the opposite may be true: if expectations are rising at a higher rate, the quality gap (see Figure 1.3) will be widening. An example of the relevance of the quality gap is the drug Viagra. Until 1998, patients' experiences with treatment for impotence and related conditions did not differ very much from their expectations, and by and large they would not have expressed particular dissatisfaction. However, following a decision to give particular patient groups restricted access to the new drug, the service provided was actually better than before. Nevertheless, because expectations had been raised (by the media rather than the NHS), many patients – and indeed

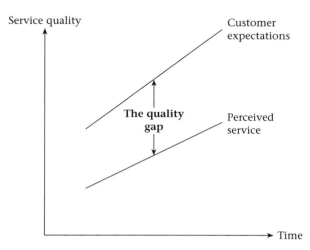

Figure 1.3 The quality gap

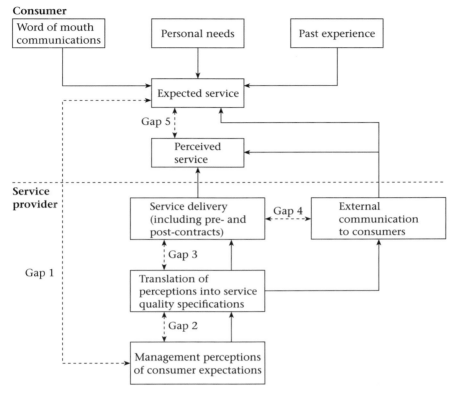

Figure 1.4   Parasuraman *et al.*'s gap analysis model (1985)

people who had not previously indicated that they might need such treatment – expressed dissatisfaction with the service provided.

   This gap between what customers expect and the quality of the service as they perceive it has been analysed by Parasuraman *et al.* (1985) (see Figure 1.4). This analysis, which builds on the same authors' discussion of perceptions and expectations described on page 24, is very useful for deciding how best to improve quality. The gap analysis model provides a framework for investigating deficiencies in service quality. Parasuraman *et al.* define service quality to be a function of the gap between customers' expectations of a service before they receive it and their perceptions of the service that they subsequently receive. This gap (Gap 5 in Figure 1.4) will always exist when a service is perceived as being of poor quality, and the model helps to identify what causes this mismatch between perceptions and expectations. Is it because management did not understand customer requirements and expectations (Gap 1)? Or perhaps management knew what the customer wanted but did not translate these requirements into specifications (Gap 2)? Maybe the specifications were fine from the customers' point of view, but the service that was actually delivered did not match these specifications (Gap 3). Alternatively, the main problem might be that communications to customers raised expectations which were not delivered (Gap 4). Let us look at these gaps in more detail.

- *Gap 1: consumer expectations vs. management perceptions of consumer expectations.* This gap arises when service managers do not understand certain aspects of what patients and service users require. For example, a doctor in one hospital informed a woman that her husband's test results were not good and that there was nothing that could be done for him medically – and then rather abruptly left the ward. The doctor did not appreciate that the woman needed her to repeat the statement several times, and in different ways, for the message to sink in. Also, the woman needed to know what nursing care her husband would require.
- *Gap 2: management perceptions vs. service quality specifications actually set.* In other cases managers may know what the customer requires, but they do not always translate this into appropriate service specifications. This may be because of a lack of resources, organizational constraints, or insufficient management commitment to a service culture. It may also be due to management regarding some consumer expectations as unreasonable or unrealistic. For example, a social services manager may know that a particular family might expect a social worker to visit them within one week, but they might set a target of one month for families with what they term non-urgent needs.
- *Gap 3: service quality specifications vs. actual service delivery.* The service performance gap occurs when the service that is delivered is different from management's service specifications. This can be due to individual members of staff being either unable or unwilling to perform at a desired level, which can in turn be due to poor training or poor morale. This gap can also result from the specifications being unrealistic given the equipment and staffing provided. In the social services example above, Gap 3 could occur if the manager specified that all such visits should take place within one week, but the allocated social worker had an urgent investigation and had to cancel the visit.
- *Gap 4: actual service delivery vs. external communications about the service.* Here what is said about the service in advertising and other communications to customers differs from the service that is delivered. For example, a GP surgery may publicize a new foot clinic, but if patients subsequently find out that they have to wait three months to get an appointment, they are unlikely to be satisfied. If expectations are too high, the service may receive a poor quality rating, so it is better to under-promise and over-deliver. This gap is particularly important when considering external communications with patients, service users and other groups. Since organizations in health and social care are very much in the public arena,

Table 1.8 Quality gaps

Gap	Description	Attitude	Rail example
1	Customers' expectations not understood by management.	There's no point asking our customers what they want – we know best.	A rail operator who does not appreciate the need to inform passengers about the reasons for a delay.
2	Management knows what the customer wants, but doesn't translate this into appropriate service specifications.	Customers have told us what they want but there's no way we're going to provide that!	Management realizes that passengers do not want to be kept waiting at the ticket office but does not provide enough staff.
3	Service delivery does not meet the specifications set due to poor training, poor morale or inadequate resources.	I know what we staff are supposed to do – but why should I bother?	A ticket inspector who is rude to customers even though they may be told to be polite.
4	Customer expectations are raised unrealistically.	Tell the customers we offer the best service. It may not be true but at least it gets them through the door.	A company that advertises a reduced price ticket if purchased seven days in advance, but does not inform passengers that they only offer a limited number of these.

they are constantly under pressure to give the message that people want to hear. However, if the message creates unrealistic expectations that do not match the reality of patients' or service users' experience, people's perceptions of the quality of service will be negative.

- *Gap 5: expected service vs. perceived service.* As mentioned earlier, Gap 5 always exists when a service is perceived as being of poor quality and is always caused by at least one of Gaps 1, 2, 3 or 4.

To conclude this chapter, Table 1.8 shows the staff and management attitudes lurking behind Gaps 1–4 of Parasuraman *et al.*'s model and also gives an example for a rail operator.

CHAPTER two

Quality management

Quality control, assurance and management

There are many quality 'buzzwords' going round both in health and social care, and in the wider business world. These include quality control, quality assurance, quality management and total quality management (TQM). To some extent these terms are used interchangeably (i.e. incorrectly!) but it is important to understand their meaning and their differences.

Definitions of each of these approaches are given in the middle columns of Table 2.1. These approaches describe something that is almost sequential. Quality control is often the first step towards quality assurance, and for quality assurance to work effectively it needs the commitment of managers and the involvement of staff, which is more like quality management. Finally, if quality management is implemented throughout the organization it is moving towards TQM.

The right-hand column of Table 2.1 shows how the definitions might apply to a clinical laboratory. Double checking that a clinical test has been analysed correctly would be quality control, while feeding back information on quality problems which are found in the checking process and changing the procedures to reduce the number of incorrect assessments is quality assurance. However, the source of many of the problems arising could include lack of staff motivation, training and involvement, poor communication with other professionals and poor leadership. Addressing those problems within the laboratory is quality management. The testing laboratory will of course typically be in a hospital setting and some of the problems users encounter will not be under the control of the laboratory staff (e.g. car parking, signage, referring processes). TQM across the whole hospital, and possibly other health and social care services, would be needed to address these areas.

Table 2.1 Approaches to quality improvement

Approach	Definition	Clinical test example
Quality control	Controlling and monitoring processes to produce quality products and services.	Double checking that a clinical test has been analysed correctly.
Quality assurance	Also concerned with the prevention of quality problems through planned and systematic activities including documentation, training, and reviewing the process.	Feeding back information on quality problems which are found in the checking process and changing the procedures to reduce the number of incorrect assessments.
Quality management	This focuses also on the management and people issues involved in achieving real and lasting quality improvement.	Addressing, within the laboratory, issues such as poor motivation, training, staff involvement, communication and leadership.
TQM	A management philosophy which applies to all parts of the organization.	Going beyond the laboratory to address the problems users encounter not just in the laboratory but in the whole hospital and referring agencies.

Quality control and quality assurance are very important aspects of quality management. These areas are particularly strong in social care where staff supervision and staff development are widespread. Indeed, as the Department of Health (2001b) points out 'for professionals with a social care background, it is easy to forget that such systems are not widespread outside this field'. However, practice varies on whether feedback from supervision results in changed policies (in which case it would be quality assurance) or just ensures that practices are carried out correctly (quality control).

Quality management builds on quality assurance but also addresses the management and people issues involved in achieving lasting quality improvement. The difference between quality management and TQM is that the latter involves working with partner organizations to ensure quality for its service users throughout the whole organization, rather than just in one area. In this book we will use 'quality management' as an 'umbrella' term which includes quality management, TQM, continuous improvement and similar initiatives.

Joss and Kogan (1995) identify three types of quality initiative: technical quality, generic quality and systemic quality (see Table 2.2). A consultant

Table 2.2   Types of quality initiative

Type	Definition
Technical quality	Concerned with the technical-professional content of work within a given area.
Generic quality	Concerned with meeting and following generally agreed or imposed standards on those aspects of quality which involve interpersonal relationships including civility, punctuality and respect for others.
Systemic quality	Concerned with making sure that the whole organization works as an integrated whole.

making a decision on whether to change over to a more modern piece of equipment to improve diagnosis will be primarily concerned with technical quality. An outpatient manager who is trying to decide how to respond to patient complaints on the comfort of the seating and on the attitudes of certain staff will be focusing mainly on generic quality, while a supplies manager who is trying to keep costs down while making sure that no one goes short of any vital equipment will be concentrating mainly on systemic issues.

Most quality initiatives in health and social care are of the technical and generic kind. Carr and Littman (1993) describe this as the 'spotty quality approach'. However, for quality approaches to make a significant impact on all aspects of the organization's activities, they need to be of the systemic type. TQM and the Excellence Model (see Chapter 4) are examples of systemic approaches. In health care, Clinical Governance is also intended to be a systemic initiative.

Total quality management (TQM)

TQM has gained wide coverage and many reported successes in a wide variety of organizations in the private and public sectors. However, there have been failures too in other organizations who have adopted the TQM approach because it seemed the right buzzword, but have ignored many of its features. TQM is not a bolt-on method that allows managers to continue as before, but with this extra 'tool' called TQM. It requires them to rethink their entire management strategy. It is not possible to have TQM and continue to shout at staff about things beyond their control, or make cuts in staff or services for short-term financial reasons without considering the impact on patients and service users. Everything needs to be integrated to ensure quality throughout the organization. A useful definition of TQM is: 'TQM is an ongoing process, requiring commitment from top management and involving everyone in the organization, to meet the requirements of service users and other stakeholders while keeping costs to a minimum'. The definition is expanded in Table 2.3.

Table 2.3 TQM

Total	Organization-wide, not in pockets.
Quality	Meeting the requirements and expectations of service users and other stakeholders while keeping costs to a minimum.
Management	An ongoing process with commitment from top management.

An alternative definition is given by Øvretveit (1997): 'a comprehensive strategy of organisational and attitude change, for enabling personnel to learn and use quality methods, in order to reduce costs and meet the requirements of patients and other customers'.

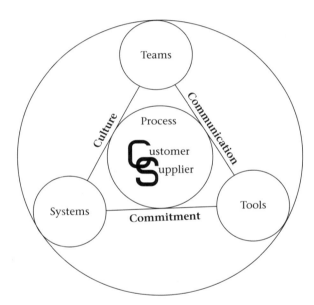

Figure 2.1 Oakland's model of TQM
Source: Oakland (2000: 181).

Oakland's model

A useful model of TQM is that of John Oakland (2000), shown in Figure 2.1. The core of TQM is the customer-supplier interface where the processes must be managed. This includes all internal and external customers and partners who need to work together to provide a seamless service for patients, users and carers. Next comes what Oakland calls the 'soft' outcomes of TQM: culture, communication and commitment – known as the 'three Cs'. These provide the foundations of the model. Surrounding the process core are some 'hard' management necessities:

- *Systems*: perhaps based on ISO9000 or some other international standard.
- *Tools*: statistical and other tools to analyse and improve the process.
- *Teams*: quality improvement teams, quality circles etc.

One of the uses of this model is in assessing an organization's quality improvement programme. Do staff work together to provide a seamless service for users? Does the organization address the three Cs above? Does it have appropriate systems and processes in place? Does it make use of statistical and other quality management tools and is there sufficient emphasis on partnership and team working?

Core concepts of TQM

TQM is based on a number of core concepts:

- commitment and example from top management;
- an organization-wide commitment to quality;
- focus on patients and service users;
- a participative environment and teamwork;
- pursuit of continuous improvement;
- quality systems;
- quality suppliers and partners.

Commitment and example from top management

A sustained, coordinated approach to improving quality requires complete commitment from top management, otherwise it will be impossible to persuade employees that quality is being taken seriously. Quality must not be seen as an added extra which can be dispensed with when new pressures arrive. All experience of quality improvement indicates that continuing commitment is vital to achieve real and sustained improvements in quality.

There are many examples of quality improvement programmes which have lacked this commitment from the top. The following example is typical:

> The chief executive gets everyone together, explains why quality is all-important and that they must improve their service to customers. Quality circles are set up and posters are put up everywhere with statements like 'Business is like tennis, if you don't serve well you lose'. One quality circle comes up with an idea that, for a modest investment, will both improve the service and lead to reduced operating costs. However, the senior manager responsible says that there are no funds available for the project.

There are a number of ways for senior managers to show commitment. These include the following:

- Being on hand when problems arise and providing a lead which indicates concern for patients and service users, while supporting staff in their efforts to improve quality.
- Making an effective contribution at quality presentations and open days.
- Getting involved in quality training days and being prepared to answer difficult questions, particularly about quality and resources.
- Chairing top quality committees rather than delegating responsibility.
- Recognizing and celebrating quality improvements.

An organization-wide commitment to quality

Quality improvement must involve everyone in the organization. It cannot be delegated to a specialist group of people. It has to be organization-wide. It is not sufficient to have an enlightened quality philosophy in, say, the X-ray department if patients are delayed in other parts of the hospital before they get to X-ray. Similarly, excellent work with families with children who need foster care will not provide a quality service if selection and support for foster carers is poor.

Joss and Kogan (1995) stressed the importance of this in their study of a number of TQM-based initiatives in the NHS. They concluded that one of the main lessons from their study was that medical staff, clinical directors, nurses etc., at all levels of the organization, should be involved right from the start. They also noted that the chief executive at one of the few sites in their sample that had managed to secure the cooperation of significant numbers of doctors said he put his success down to his long-standing and cordial relationships with the medical director and the chair of medical audit.

Focus on patients and service users

The quality philosophy of the organization should be focused on patients and service users. Identifying the needs of different groups of patients or service users and organizing the service around those needs is the essence of quality management. This includes making sure that staff develop people skills, including training where appropriate, and that such skills are valued. It is also important to make sure that processes are geared to patients and service users.

I can recall one example of excellent practice when I went to hospital for a very minor 30-second operation. Despite this, I still had my anxieties: would it hurt, were there any risks attached? To my delight, the doctor introduced herself, set me at my ease, listened to my concerns, seemed in no hurry to rush me through and did not make me feel stupid about worrying about something so minor.

Another example is a single father of a boy with multiple disabilities, John, who subsequently died. The father reported having received considerable help and support from the social worker, not only when John was alive but also after he died. The social worker had become one of the few people who knew his son very well and he would have been even more devastated without her occasional visits after John's death.

A participative environment and teamwork

Getting staff to participate in quality initiatives is the key to improving quality. It is the staff of the organization who deliver quality. Encouraging positive attitudes among staff towards the customer, providing the right training for them, making it clear what is expected of them and listening to their needs and ideas for improvement will set the service well on the way to making real improvements in quality. As Dilly Millward, former Director of Nursing and Quality Assurance at Hastings and Rother NHS Trust, says, 'The best marketing tool any organization has is its staff. If you do not involve, motivate and commit them to your value system then you will never get total quality and customer service'.

Pursuit of continuous improvement

This means constantly finding out whether customers are happy with the service provided and, if not, analysing the problem to see how the service can be improved. However, the emphasis should not be on apportioning blame to individuals but on finding out what can be done to prevent the problem recurring, or at least to reduce its frequency as much as possible. Managers, professionals and other staff should take note of the following statement from the report on *Best Value in Local Government* from the joint Scottish Office/Convention of Scottish Local Authorities (COSLA) task force (Scottish Office/COSLA 1997): 'Where councils discover that their services fail to achieve satisfactory performance, then continuous improvement requires that they take action. For many councils this will require some investigation to identify the reason for the discrepancy, and appropriate action to close the gap'.

Quality systems

A positive attitude to patients and service users is a vital ingredient of quality management, but it is not sufficient without proper quality systems. In social care, for example, it is well known that appropriate systems are needed for allocating new referrals and documenting a visit or meeting with a service user. Otherwise there may well be delays in visiting the service user or confusion if another member of staff picks up a case without adequate information. In each case, despite positive attitudes of staff, service users will get a poor deal.

Everyone needs to appreciate the vital contribution of effective and efficient systems and processes, and managers need to understand how to go about improving and developing them. This can only happen if the culture is one that sees the whole organization as a dynamic entity depending on the success and coordination of all its component systems. The old view (and sometimes the current reality) of the organization as a collection of independent departments, often in conflict, has to be replaced. Management has to present a vision of cooperation, communication and interdepartmental teamwork.

Quality suppliers and partners

In any organization, quality depends not only on the organization itself but also on its suppliers and partners. A key task of quality improvement is to ensure that suppliers and partners are providing the appropriate goods and services to meet the needs of the organization and its service users.

The Best Value initiative addresses this aspect of quality explicitly. A quality service organization cannot rely on suppliers who simply meet minimum standards at the lowest cost. Best Value aims to give organizations flexibility in their choice of suppliers and enable them to take both quality and cost into account. Just as importantly, it also gives the message to potential suppliers or contractors that the organization is concerned about quality and that they need to pay more than lip-service to quality if they are to win the contract.

It is also important to have very good working relationships with, and commitment from, partners across organizational boundaries. Many children with suspected non-accidental injuries first come to the attention of a social services department via staff in schools or in the local hospital. Any delays due to school or hospital staff not notifying social services early enough may have serious consequences for the child.

Quality initiatives in health and social care

While quality has always been a major concern in health and social care, in the UK the term TQM did not begin to be used in these sectors until the 1980s. Following this, in the early 1990s, the Department of Health sponsored a number of pilot TQM projects. In evaluating these projects, Joss and Kogan (1995) concluded that while some sites achieved major improvements, most did not fully commit themselves to TQM and the benefits varied considerably.

Perhaps partly because of these pilots, TQM did not get a good name within the NHS, but as in the commercial world there can be a considerable gap between the claim to be using TQM and actual implementation. What carries a TQM label is all too often far from 'total', has little impact on service quality and is managed only in the sense that it is 'stage-managed', giving the impression of change where little of significance is actually happening.

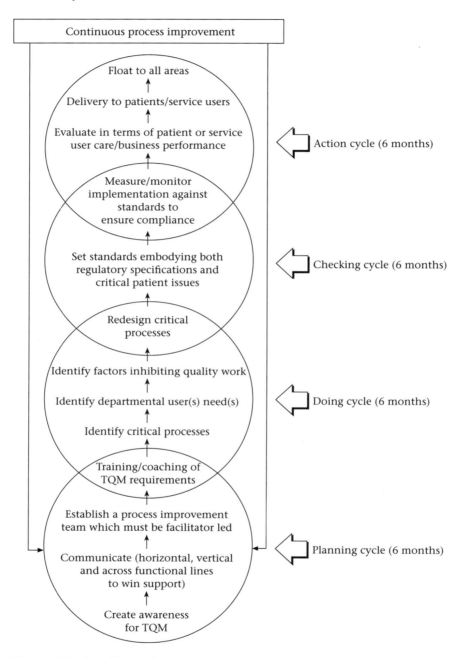

Figure 2.2 Spiral loop of a systems model for TQM implementation in the NHS
Source: Haigh and Morris (2001).

Based on their analysis from their analysis of TQM projects in health services, Nwabuese and Kanji (1997) proposed the model shown in Figure 2.2 for the implementation of TQM. This model shows the steps required in each of Deming's (1986) four phases of his cycle for continuous improvement: plan, do, check, act (see page 55). Nwabuese and Kanji (1997) cite the factors listed below, among others, as being critical to the success of TQM:

- leadership and commitment from top management;
- adopting a holistic approach by involving everyone;
- communicating extensively across functional and directorate lines;
- identifying key processes, redesigning them when necessary while allowing ownership of processes by the people who work on them;
- instituting honesty, allowing room for staff to learn from their mistakes;
- instituting a robust system of monitoring and measurement of critical processes and outcomes.

Organizations in health and social care have always been concerned about the quality of their services and there has been a wide variety of initiatives over a long period spanning the areas of quality control, quality assurance and quality management. However, at no time has the number of quality-related initiatives been greater than at present and staff are in danger of initiative overload.

This section discusses the following quality-related initiatives used by organizations in health and social care: the NHS Plan, Clinical Governance, Best Value, *Modernizing Social Services*, *A Quality Strategy for Social Care*, Investors in People and Charter Mark. Three others (ISO9000, the Excellence Model and the Balanced Scorecard) are considered in Chapters 3, 4 and 9 respectively.

The NHS Plan

The NHS Plan is by far the most ambitious and comprehensive attempt at improving quality in health and social care in the UK. It is a long-term plan involving investment by the government, changed methods of working and a change of culture. The vision of the NHS Plan is 'to offer people fast and convenient care delivered to a consistently high standard. Services will be available when people require them, tailored to their individual needs' (National Health Service 2000).

The core principles of the NHS Plan are as follows:

- The NHS will provide a universal service for all, based on clinical need not ability to pay.
- The NHS will provide a comprehensive range of services.
- The NHS will shape its services around the needs and preferences of individual patients, their families and their carers.

- The NHS will respond to the different needs of different populations.
- The NHS will work continuously to improve quality services and to minimize errors.
- The NHS will support and value its staff.
- Public funds for health care will be devoted solely to NHS patients.
- The NHS will work together with others to ensure a seamless service for patients.
- The NHS will help keep people healthy and work to reduce health inequalities.
- The NHS will respect the confidentiality of individual patients and provide open access to information about services, treatment and performance.

The NHS Plan is wide-ranging and includes investments in extra beds and hospitals, more staff, better child care, changed systems based on the NHS as a 'high trust organization', redesigning care around patients, effective team working, more patient choice and information, cutting waiting times for treatment, improving health and reducing inequality and providing dignity, security and independence in old age.

The Plan has implications for social care as well as health. In particular it aims to ensure that social services work seamlessly with health services to provide integrated care, particularly for older people and people with mental health problems. Local authorities will work alongside primary care and health authorities to put in place rapid response teams to avoid unnecessary hospital admission, intensive rehabilitation services, short-term nursing care and supported accommodation to aid recuperation and integrated home care teams. The Plan also provides flexibility to pool budgets across social and health services to aid partnership working.

It is interesting to note that despite the only partial success of the TQM pilots in the early 1990s, lessons do appear to have been learnt. In particular, the Plan has attempted to address each of the factors cited by Nwabuese and Kanji at least to some extent. The government and the NHS have provided some leadership themselves, with some commitment in terms of increased resources. There is more patient and carer involvement, greater involvement of clinicians, more emphasis on certain key processes and a commitment to create a climate of openness. They also propose to improve the monitoring of critical processes through the National Performance Assessment Framework. This of course is only a start – there is a vast amount of work still to be done – but it is a start nevertheless.

The Plan is ambitious in scope and cannot succeed without the commitment of staff both within the NHS and in partner organizations. As Tony Blair says in the introduction to the Plan: 'It will of course take time to achieve it all. But taken as a whole, it does offer the genuine opportunity to re-build the NHS for the 21st century, true to its priorities but radically reformed in their implementation (National Health Service 2000).

Clinical Governance

Clinical Governance is a major plank of the government's strategy on quality in health. Many previous initiatives in health skirted round the main clinical areas of the NHS, looking at waiting times and design of waiting rooms but avoiding the core service provided. Clinical Governance is a systematic approach to help clinicians and others assess, improve and monitor the quality of these core services. Its aim, according to Henry Stahr, Excellence Development Manager at Salford Royal Hospitals NHS Trust, is 'changing the culture of the whole organization so that quality of patient care is the driving force for all'.

Clinical Governance is 'a framework through which NHS organisations are accountable for continuously improving the quality of their services and safeguarding high standards of care by creating an environment in which excellence in care will flourish' (NHS Executive 1999a). Its main components are as follows:

- Clear lines of responsibility and accountability for the overall quality of clinical care.
- A comprehensive programme of quality improvement systems (including clinical audit, supporting and applying evidence-based practice, implementing clinical standards and guidelines, workforce planning and development).
- Education and training plans.
- Clear policies aimed at managing risk.
- Integrated procedures for all professional groups to identify and remedy poor performance.

The Commission for Health Improvement's (CHI) model for Clinical Governance (see Figure 2.3) shows the key role of information in supporting Clinical Governance. Without relevant information, it is impossible to evaluate possible service improvements and strategies. The model also illustrates how 'effective clinical governance depends on a culture of continuous learning, innovation and development and will improve patients' experience of care and treatment in hospital' (Bevan and Bawden 2001).

The aim of Clinical Governance is to encourage good performance, rather than concentrating on those who are performing relatively poorly. Peter Homa, chief executive of the CHI, says: 'Everyone knows that standards vary across the NHS. CHI will raise standards across the board by highlighting excellence and not just pulling its punches where improvement is needed'.

In implementing Clinical Governance, Dillon (2001) suggests that clinical staff and others should ask themselves four questions:

- What do we expect of ourselves?
- What tests are we going to apply to our performance from which we can draw conclusions about the quality of what we do?
- What benchmarks adequately describe our definition of a good standard of care?
- What would we expect for ourselves as patients using our own services?

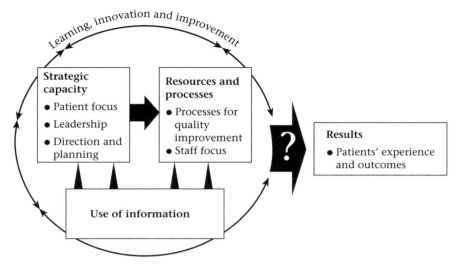

Figure 2.3 The Commission for Health Improvement's model for
Clinical Governance
Source: Bevan and Bawden (2001).

Best Value

Best Value is not specifically a quality management programme, although
improving the quality of services is one of its main aims. It is a central
government initiative requiring local authorities to produce a series of best
value reviews on the services they provide. The main aims of these reviews
are to improve services for individuals, to enable authorities to shape better
services, to promote better standards and improve the management of practice, and to secure better value for money. They are intended to be wide-
ranging, focusing on quality and value for money, with increased emphasis
on partnerships with private industry, the voluntary sector and other public
bodies.

Best Value reviews need to address the following key questions:

- Why are we delivering this service and what is it meant to achieve?
- What do the public want from us?
- How do we compare to other councils or service providers?
- How do other councils provide this service?
- Are there other agencies or organizations that could deliver this service
  for us?
- Is the service we provide competitive and as efficient as it could be?

A key aspect is replacing compulsive competitive tendering, which required
councils to choose suppliers who meet minimum standards at the lowest
cost. Best Value aims to give organizations flexibility in their choice of

suppliers and enable them to take both quality and cost into account in awarding contracts. There is also a political agenda concerned with making greater use of the private sector.

In carrying out a Best Value review, organizations need to take account of the 'four Cs':

- *Challenge* why and how a service is provided. This aspect is perhaps the most crucial. Not only does the organization need to decide the purpose of the service and whether there are alternative ways of meeting people's requirements, it also needs to challenge whether the service is best provided in-house or by others.
- *Compare* against relevant performance indicators. Performance measurement and monitoring is a key element of Best Value. Organizations will need to collect information and set targets on a range of national Best Value performance indicators and benchmark against others in the public and private sectors.
- *Consult* with a wide range of local and other interested parties. Developing partnerships – with service users and others with an interest in the service (e.g. parents of schoolchildren) local taxpayers, other public bodies, the voluntary and private sectors – is another theme of Best Value.
- *Compete* to ensure competitiveness. This involves 'fair and open competition wherever practical as a means of securing efficient and effective services' (Department of the Environment, Transport and the Regions 1999).

Best Value has a number of aspects in common with quality management – a service user/citizen focus and an emphasis on continuous improvement, value for money and performance measurement. However it is noticeably lacking on the softer aspects of TQM: culture, communication and commitment (the three Cs of Oakland's model, see p. 39). There is also no real model indicating how Best Value can be achieved. The Excellence Model (see Chapter 4) on the other hand does provide such a framework and several local authorities (notably Cheshire, Warwickshire, Devon and Hertfordshire) have used this model to support Best Value.

Modernising Social Services

The White Paper, *Modernising Social Services*, launched in 1998 (Department of Health 1998c) covered a number of quality-related programmes including proposals for better support for adults and the Quality Protects programme, which aimed to transform children's social services.

For adults the main priorities for improvement are concerned with promoting independence (aimed at helping people who need care to have as independent and active a life as is possible); improving consistency, setting national objectives for social services and ensuring fair access; and providing convenient, user-centred services, making services easier to use and more tailored to individual needs.

Quality Protects is a government programme concerned with effective protection, better quality care and improved life chances for children. It has a number of objectives:

- ensuring stable, secure, safe and effective care for all children;
- protecting children from abuse and neglect;
- better life chances for children in need: good education, health care and social care for all children;
- good life chances for children in care: good education, health care and social care;
- enabling young people leaving care to live successful adult lives;
- meeting the needs of disabled children and their families;
- better assessment leading to better services;
- actively involving users and carers;
- using regulation to protect children;
- making sure that child care workers are fit for the job;
- making best use of resources: choice, effectiveness and value for money.

A Quality Strategy for Social Care

While *Modernising Social Services* focused on changes in systems and structures, the publication *A Quality Strategy for Social Care* (Department of Health 2000b) looked at 'reforms needed in working practices, local management and training in order to drive up the quality of social services in England'. There are three main parts to this strategy:

- The new Social Care Institute for Excellence. This aims to improve the evidence base about what works best in social care, to improve quality and to stimulate change.
- A new quality framework. This addresses accountability arrangements for councillors and senior staff, a commitment to staff development, an emphasis on partnership working and assessment of the performance of local councils.
- Proposals for improved workforce training, including social work education and training for front-line managers.

Investors in People

Investors in People (IiP) is a national standard for effective investment in the training and development of people in order to achieve organizational goals. IiP has been used by a large number of organizations in health and social care, many of whom have achieved the standard. Smith (1998) believes that 'IiP is a great hope for many in the social care sector offering the promise of aligning personal and organisational objectives and providing proper staff development opportunities'. IiP is based on four key principles:

- a commitment to develop all employees;
- a regular review of the training and development needs of employers and a plan to meet those needs;
- action to train and develop individuals throughout their improvement;
- the measurement of the organization's success in using its investment in training and development effectively.

While Investors in People does address these issues well, there is a danger that organizations may see attainment of the standard as an indicator that they have effective human resource management processes. There is however much more to human resources than training and development. Developing a service-user focused culture, team working and empowerment are other key aspects (see Chapter 6).

Charter Mark

Charter Mark is a government award scheme introduced in 1992 to recognize and encourage excellence in public service delivery. Applicants need to demonstrate that their performance satisfies set criteria, and if so they get the Charter Mark award. It was relaunched in 1998 following an extensive consultation exercise with greater emphasis on quality, effectiveness, responsiveness and coordination.

Charter Mark focuses on the outcome for the customer, rather than the management processes used by an organization to deliver a service. If an organization reaches the Charter Mark standard, it shows that it puts its users first and delivers a first-class service. Unlike some schemes it is not 'paper hungry' – a 12-page application form together with no more than one box file of supplementary evidence is all that is required.

Charter Mark is based on 'ten principles of public service which represent the Government's vision of what every public service should be striving to achieve and by which Charter Mark applications are judged' (Cabinet Office 1999). These are as follows:

- *Set standards of service* that users can expect, monitor and review performance and publish the results, following independent validation wherever possible.
- *Be open and provide full information* clearly and effectively in plain language, to help people using public services and provide full information about services, their cost and how well they perform.
- *Consult and involve* present and potential users of public services, as well as those who work in them, and use their views to improve the service provided.
- *Encourage access and the promotion of choice*: make services easily available to everyone who needs them, including using new technology to the full and offering choice wherever possible.

- *Treat all people fairly*, respect their privacy and dignity, be helpful and courteous and pay particular attention to those with special needs.
- *Put things right when they go wrong*, quickly and effectively, learn from complaints and have a clear, well publicized and easy-to-use complaints procedure with independent review wherever possible.
- *Use resources effectively* to provide best value for taxpayers and users.
- *Innovate and improve*: always look for ways to improve the services and facilities offered.
- *Work with other providers* to ensure that services are simple to use, effective, coordinated and deliver a better service to the user.
- *Provide user satisfaction*: Show that your users are satisfied with the quality of service they are receiving.

The Philosophies of Deming, Juran and Crosby

Deming, Juran and Crosby are perhaps the best known of the many quality 'gurus' who have contributed well to our knowledge and understanding of quality. Although they mainly addressed the needs of the private sector, and manufacturing in particular, the basic principles apply to all organizations.

W. Edwards Deming

One of the original quality pioneers, Dr Deming is perhaps the most well known of the quality gurus. An American who was not listened to in his own country, Deming went to Japan where he greatly assisted the Japanese in their remarkable improvements in quality since the 1950s.

Originally trained as a statistician, much of Deming's earlier work was in the area of statistical process control. He was one of the first people to apply this in a service environment, using it in preparation for the 1940 US census. Routine clerical operations were improved in this way, leading to sixfold productivity improvements in some areas.

He was then asked to teach his methods to US industrialists. However, Deming's influence in his own country was limited, particularly in the boom market after the war where everything that was produced was sold with or without quality control. As Deming recalls (Mann 1985), 'The courses were well-received by engineers, but management paid no attention to them. Management did not understand that they had to get behind improvement of quality and carry out their obligations from the top down . . . Changing the process is management's responsibility. And we failed to teach them that'.

After the war Deming went to Japan, originally as an adviser to the Japanese census, and by 1950 his ideas were well received by the top management of Sony, Nissan, Mitsubishi, Toyota and other companies soon to be well known in the West. His success was such that in 1960 the Japanese emperor awarded him the Second Order of the Sacred Treasure for his role in

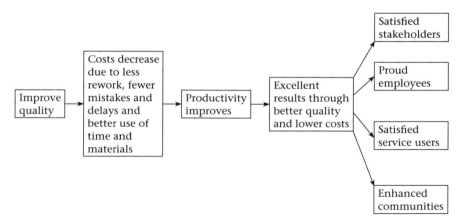

Figure 2.4 Deming's chain reaction

the creation of modern Japanese industrial success. Deming's contribution at this stage was mainly to cut through the academic theory of statistical methods and 'present the ideas in a simple way which could be meaningful right down to production worker levels' (Hutchings 1990: 77).

Deming's chain reaction

Deming's general philosophy is summarized in his 'chain reaction'. This is shown in Figure 2.4, although the four boxes on the right-hand side have been added, showing the benefits more clearly. The chain reaction summarizes the discussion in Chapter 1 on the costs of quality. When quality is improved costs decrease – for example, because processes are performed right first time, there are fewer delays and fewer complaints to deal with. This improves productivity and the organization can then produce excellent results through better quality and lower costs. This leads to satisfied service users and other stakeholders, proud employees and enhanced communities.

Understanding variation

Deming once said, 'If I had to reduce my message to just a few words, I'd say it all had to do with reducing variation'. By this he meant that if variation is reduced then the reliability, dependability, predictability and consistency of products and services will all improve. Reducing variation will therefore improve quality and reduce costs.

Variation is widely misunderstood. Suppose the number of patients treated in a particular month is less than in the preceding month. The reaction of many managers and professionals would be to imply that performance has got worse and that something needs to be done to get performance back on track. However, the correct approach is to ask *why* the number of patients treated has gone down. Is it due to random variation from month to month (e.g. the mix of patients may have changed with fewer straightforward cases), or is it due to a particular change in the policies or procedures used? If it is the former, then interfering with the system is not required and can make matters worse.

Blaming staff for variations in performance without first analysing the reasons for those variations is also very common. This is not only unjust, but is likely to be counterproductive:

> The discovery of a *special* cause of variation and its removal, are usually the responsibility of someone who is connected directly with some operation. In contrast there are *common* causes of defectives, of errors, of low rates or production, of low sales, of accidents. These are the responsibility of management. The worker at the machine can do nothing about causes common to all machines. He cannot do anything about the light, he does not purchase raw materials; the training, supervision, and the company's policies are not his.
>
> (Deming 1982: 116)

Deming encouraged managers to identify whether variability is due to:

- Special or assignable causes, including changes in the raw materials, operators and procedures used;

or

- common or unassignable causes. All of these are due to the process itself, its design and installation. Variability can be seen as random and as natural from week to week. Note 'common' is used in the sense that the causes could happen to any particular product or service, rather than that they occur frequently.

Classifying variation is an important first step in analysing variation in many performance indicators in health and social care. Analysis of hospital-acquired infection, numbers of patients with coronary heart disease receiving care within the waiting-time targets and the proportion of older people helped to live at home are just a few such examples.

Common and special cause variation in operating theatres

Nicholls *et al.* (2001) give the example of a manager reviewing the performance of an operating theatre, who may decide to analyse 'overruns' (late finishes). The manager needs an understanding of the systems and processes used in the theatre and needs to begin by apportioning any variation to either day-to-day variation or one-off sporadic, unusual events. Examples of the two types of variation are shown in Table 2.4. Nicholls *et al.* (2001) conclude

Table 2.4 Day-to-day and special cause variation in an operating theatre

Day-to-day variation	Variation due to special causes
Different patients with different problems	Lack of theatre greens (overalls) due to laundry or portering problems
Different staff with different problems, training and needs	Change in clerking procedures as a result of a new ward policy, the arrival of a new consultant or the introduction of a different surgical procedure
Different equipment	
Staff defining and measuring overruns differently	
Different protocols or techniques for the same operation	

that 'Variation in results occasioned by everyday events should be ignored – tampering with systems because of day-to-day variation only increases problems and reduces performance . . . It is variation due to . . . sporadic, unusual events which needs to be investigated'.

Deming's cycle of continuous improvement

How does Deming recommend that quality improvement should be achieved? A key aspect to this is his plan, do, check, act cycle of continuous improvement, originally developed by Shewhart (1931). Until 1990 this was known as plan, do, check and act but Deming changed the third item to *study* because with only a 'check' one might miss something. The 'PDSA' cycle is illustrated in Figure 2.5.

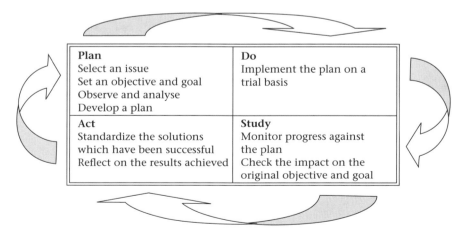

Figure 2.5 The Deming cycle of continuous improvement

The National Primary Care Development Team (2002), which has used the PDSA cycle on a number of occasions, concluded that 'testing small changes sequentially means that design problems can be detected and amended earlier rather than later, saving huge amounts of effort being put into massive change which has to be altered'. They recommend that the process should be kept simple and manageable to start with and that cycles should happen quickly: 'think in terms of a week not a month'. There is they say no wrong answer – if something works then use it.

Deming's 14 points

Deming's (1986) 14 points for senior management, which are often quoted, are aimed at helping people understand and implement the necessary transformation to a quality organization. They are as follows:

- Create and publish to all employees a statement of the aims and purposes of the company or other organization. The management must demonstrate constantly their commitment to this statement.
- Learn the new philosophy (top management and everybody).
- Understand the purpose of inspection for improvement of processes and reduction of cost.
- End the practice of awarding business on the basis of price-tag alone.
- Improve constantly and forever the system of production and service.
- Institute training.
- Teach and institute leadership.
- Drive out fear. Create trust. Create a climate for innovation.
- Optimize toward the aims and purposes of the company the efforts of teams, groups and staff areas.
- Eliminate exhortations for the workforce.
- (a) Eliminate numerical quotas for production. Instead, learn and institute methods for improvement.
  (b) Eliminate 'management by objectives'. Instead, learn the capabilities of processes and how to improve them.
- Remove barriers that rob people of pride of workmanship.
- Encourage education and self-improvement for everyone.
- Take action to accomplish the transformation.

Deming's deadly diseases

If Deming's 14 points are a directive to management telling them what to do, then his 'deadly diseases' are a list of what *not* to do. Deming (1982) tells us that the deadly diseases 'stand in the way of transformation'. Some of the deadly diseases are more specific to US industrial companies, but those that are more general include:

- a lack of constancy of purpose;
- emphasis on short-term profits etc.;
- evaluation of (individual) performance, merit rating or annual review;
- mobility of management ('job hopping');
- management by use of only visible figures with little or no consideration of other factors.

Table 2.5 shows which of the 14 points address the five deadly diseases.

Table 2.5 The five deadly diseases as related to the 14 points

Disease	Point
Lack of constancy	Constancy of purpose (1) Take action (14)
Short termism	The new philosophy (2)
Evaluation of (individual) performance	Drive out fear (8) Break down barriers (9) Eliminate arbitrary numerical targets (11)
Mobility of management	Institute leadership (7)
Use of only visible figures	Eliminate arbitrary numerical targets (11) End lowest tender contracts (4)

Source: Based on Hughes (1999).

Joseph Juran

Like Deming, Joseph Juran is an American who has taught quality principles to the Japanese since the 1950s and was a major force in their quality reorganization. His background was in the electrical industry where he did much work on the development of statistical methods for quality. His book, the *Quality Control Handbook*, published in 1951 and revised several times since then (most recently in 1988) is still a popular reference book and established his reputation.

Juran's definition of quality is 'fitness for use'. He identifies two aspects to quality: product features that meet customer needs; and freedom from deficiencies. Improvement to each aspect of quality has different effects – see Table 2.6.

Juran expresses his central message through what has become known as the 'Juran trilogy' (1986) (see Table 2.7).

Table 2.6 Effects of improved quality

	Product features that meet customer needs	*Freedom from deficiencies*
Effect of improved quality	Increased customer satisfaction Increased market share Secure premium prices Meet competition	Reduced error rates Reduced rework and waste Reduced field failures Reduced customer dissatisfaction Shortened lead times Increased yields Improved delivery performance
Major effect	On sales	On costs
Effect on costs	Usually, higher quality costs more	Usually, higher quality reduces cost

Source: Juran (1986).

Table 2.7 The Juran trilogy

Quality planning	Ensuring a process capable of meeting quality goals
Quality control	Measuring quality performance against standard and acting on any differences
Quality improvement	Finding ways to do better than standard and break through to unprecedented levels of performance

For *quality planning*, Juran's 'quality planning roadmap' involves the following steps:

- identify the target customer groups, external and internal;
- determine the needs of those customers;
- translate those needs into the language of the organization;
- design product features to meet those needs;
- develop processes capable of producing those features;
- optimize the process;
- prove that the process can produce the product under operating conditions;
- transfer the process to operations.

A key aspect of the roadmap is that there should be measurement at each stage – don't just take it on trust that the relevant stage has been reached: 'It may seem surprising that one such roadmap is so universal: that it can provide directions for planning a very wide range of products and processes. Yet such is the case and it has been field tested extensively' (Juran 1989).

The *quality control* phase involves evaluating actual performance, comparing performance to goals or standards and taking action on the differences. Measurement of quality, for example by a special sensor measuring product and process features (e.g. thickness and temperature) is crucial here.

Quality improvement (i.e. raising quality performance to unprecedented levels) takes place project by project. Juran says that the great majority of quality improvement projects have achieved success by 'fine tuning' the process rather than investing in a new process. As a rule of thumb, he states that 'any process that is already producing over 80% good work can, by fine tuning, be brought up to the high 90s without capital investment. This same avoidance of capital investment is a major reason why quality improvement has so high a return on investment' (Juran 1989).

Juran gives four steps for quality improvement:

- establish the infrastructure needed to secure annual quality improvement;
- identify the specific needs for improvement – the improvement projects;
- for each project establish a project team with clear responsibility for bringing the project to a successful conclusion;
- provide the resources, motivation and training needed by the teams to diagnose the causes, develop remedies, and establish controls to keep quality at the improved level.

Philip Crosby

One of the clearest expositions on how to tackle quality improvement which is equally applicable to service and manufacturing organizations is that of Philip Crosby. His book, *Quality Without Tears: The Art of Hassle-Free Management* (1984) identifies five symptoms of troubled organizations:

- the outgoing product or service normally contains deviations from the published, announced or agreed-upon requirements;
- the company has an extensive field service or dealer network skilled in rework and resourceful corrective action to keep the customers satisfied;
- management does not provide a clear performance standard or definition of quality, so the employees each develop their own;
- management does not know the price of non-conformance;
- management denies that it is the cause of the problem.

Crosby draws a parallel with drug abuse, where the primary symptom is also denial. It is not until their life begins to fall apart that addicts realize they can't handle it. With companies this occurs when the market share shrinks and profits disappear. Crosby invites managers to complete the following questionnaire:

	Characteristic	That's us all the way (5 points)	True to some extent (3 points)	We're not like that (1 point)
1	Our services and/or products normally contain waivers, deviations and other indications of not conforming to requirements.			
2	We have a 'fix it' oriented approach.			
3	Our employees do not know what management wants from them concerning quality.			
4	Management does not know what the price of non-conformance really is.			
5	Management believes that quality problems are caused by something other than management actions.			

Depending on the score obtained, Crosby's diagnosis is as follows:

Score	Condition	Treatment
21–25	Critical	Needs intensive care immediately
16–20	Guarded	Needs life support system
11–15	Resting	Needs medication and attention
6–10	Healing	Needs regular check-up
5	Whole	Needs counselling

Crosby has four absolutes of quality management:

- quality is conformance to requirements, not goodness;
- the system for obtaining quality is prevention, not appraisal;
- the performance standard is zero defects, not 'that's close enough';
- the measurement of quality is the price of non-conformance, not indexes.

We have dealt with the first, second and fourth absolutes already in this book. However, the third absolute – zero defects – needs some further discussion.

Zero defects

One of the key aspects of Crosby's approach is the notion of zero defects. This aspect is not always understood. What Crosby claims is that an organization should not be happy even if, say, 95 per cent of customers are satisfied with a product or service. That would be tantamount to saying that they are happy for 5 per cent of customers *not* to be satisfied. The costs of 5 per cent unsatisfied customers, including the effect of them sharing their experiences with others, would be considerable. Suppose that instead 99 per cent of customers were satisfied – should the organization be satisfied now? According to Crosby the argument is the same. They shouldn't be satisfied until they have zero defects. By this Crosby is not implying that all organizations can achieve zero defects, but he is saying that they should never be complacent.

The concept of zero defects as an attitude to quality can be illustrated by examining some statements from British Telecom (BT) shareholders in their October 1991 prospectus (British Telecom 1991) (see Table 2.8). BT's statements are in the left-hand column. The right-hand column contains an alternative view of the same results based on other figures contained in the prospectus. BT's proud statements of their quality achievements are a good example of the complacent attitude that Crosby is trying to get people to move away from. BT had, even then, made significant improvements in their quality of service. However, if their attitude to quality was effectively that 400,000 dissatisfied customers each day is acceptable (or up to 800,000 if we include those at the other end of the line!) then their attitude was a long way from one of zero defects. This also provides a word of warning when measuring quality of service – do not hide behind percentages. It is usually

Table 2.8 Attitudes to quality at British Telecom (BT)

BT's statements	Alternative view
Less than 1 call in 200 failed to get through due to network faults or congestion	400,000 telephone calls fail to get through each day due to network faults or congestion
Line faults occurred on average only about once every 5 years	There were 5 million faults on telephone lines last year alone
95% of BT's public payphones were in working order	On average nearly 5000 payphones were out of action at any one time

Source: Moullin (1999).

better to refer to number of users. A satisfaction level of 95 per cent may *sound* good, but if there are 10,000 users it means that 500 are dissatisfied. That is a lot of unsatisfied people.

Crosby's 14 points

Not to be outdone by Deming, with whom he had many disagreements, Crosby's path to quality improvement also has 14 points:

- Make it clear that management is committed to quality.
- Form quality improvement teams with representatives from each department.
- Determine where current and potential problems lie.
- Evaluate the cost of quality and explain its use as a management tool.
- Raise the quality awareness and personal concern for all employees.
- Take action to correct problems identified through previous steps.
- Establish a committee for the zero defects programme.
- Train supervisors to actively carry out their part of the quality improvement programme.
- Hold a 'zero defects day' so that all employees realize there has been a change.
- Encourage individuals to establish improvement goals for themselves and their groups.
- Encourage employees to communicate to management the obstacles they face in attaining their improvement goals.
- Recognize and appreciate those who participate.
- Establish quality councils to communicate on a regular basis.
- Do it all over again to emphasize that the quality improvement programme never ends.

It is interesting to compare this list with Deming's 14 points. Both have been well received and followed in all sectors of the economy. My own feeling is that Deming's list shows better what to get rid of, while Crosby's is more helpful in saying what actually should be done.

The three gurus compared

To summarize this section and conclude this chapter, it is useful to compare the views of Deming, Juran and Crosby – Table 2.9.

Table 2.9 The three gurus compared

	Deming	Juran	Crosby
Definition of quality	A predictable degree of uniformity and dependability at low cost and suited to the market	Fitness for use	Conformance to requirements
Performance standard	Quality has many 'scales' Use statistics to measure performance Critical of zero defects	Avoid campaigns to 'do perfect work'	Zero defects
General approach	Reduce variability by continuous improvement Cease mass inspection	General management approach to quality	Prevention not inspection
Statistical process control (SPC)	Statistical methods of quality control must be used	Recommends SPC but warns that it can lead to a 'tool driven' approach	Rejects statistically acceptable levels of quality
Improvement basis	Continuous to reduce variation Eliminate goals without methods	Project by project team approach Set goals	A 'process' not a programme Improvement goals
Teamwork	Employee participation in decision making Break down barriers between departments	Team and quality circle approach	Quality improvement teams Quality councils
Costs of quality	No optimum – continuous improvement	Quality is not free – there is an optimum	Cost of non-conformance

CHAPTER three

Quality standards and quality systems

Developing and monitoring service standards is an important part of quality management. Without quality standards and measurement of performance against these standards, it is difficult to ensure that a quality improvement programme is working effectively. It is also difficult to make sure that quality improvements happen in all areas of the organization, not just those where the staff happen to be enthusiastic. There is also 'a need for standards as benchmarks so that we can move to evidence-based practice and the measurement of performance' (National Institute for Social Work 1999).

Setting service standards

Setting service standards is one of the keys to successful quality improvement. By setting a standard for an activity an organization is:

- explicitly stating its view of the requirements of patients, service users and other stakeholders;
- indicating that this view is open to question by users and staff;
- communicating to staff that it believes that this area is important;
- establishing the minimum to be achieved now.

Service standards are sometimes introduced without real commitment to quality from senior managers and without a real understanding of what customers require and expect. Unless standards are implemented as part of quality management, comparatively few benefits will result. The framework in Figure 3.1 shows how standards should be implemented. The framework illustrates that commitment to quality and teamwork, two of the cornerstones of quality management, are vital for quality standards to work effectively.

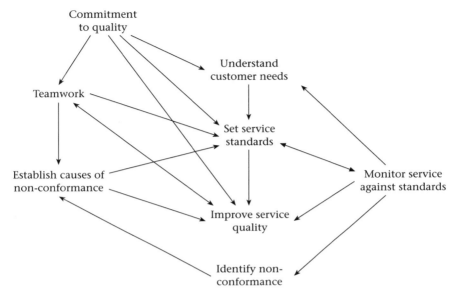

Figure 3.1 The cycle of continual quality improvement
Source: Moullin (1995).

Standards need to be based on an understanding of customer requirements and expectations. Once standards are set, steps need to be taken to identify improvements that need to be made to meet the standards. Monitoring the service provided against the standard and establishing the causes of non-conformances is also vital. As quality improves, teamwork and motivation should also improve. Things will not stand still. Customer expectations will rise and standards may be set higher still. The cycle continues and the reward for staff is being part of an organization which gives good service to patients and service users, giving rise to staff satisfaction and pride in their work.

What is a standard?

One way of visualizing the role of service standards in quality management is shown in Figure 3.2. The standard is the chock that prevents the quality of service ball falling down the hill. However, the aim is to push the ball to the top of the hill. Once the organization has achieved the current standard, it needs to push the ball further up the hill and replace the chock at a higher level. This process continues until the ball reaches the top of the hill and customers' requirements are fully met. But even when the top of the hill is reached, there will be another hill. The process is never-ending and is one of continual improvement.

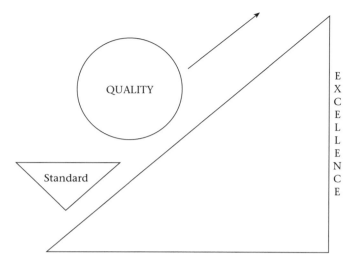

Figure 3.2 The 'ball on the hill'
Source: Koch (1991).

As an example, an outpatient clinic has a standard that patients will be seen within 30 minutes of their appointment time. The chock is currently at 30 minutes but to achieve real excellence it needs to be moved nearer the top of the hill by resetting the standard to a shorter waiting time. Another example is a breast screening service in one authority whose service standards include those shown below. Here too the standards reflect the authority's view on what can realistically be achieved. Any improvement in these times would, however, have a marked impact on reducing anxiety for those with or without a cancerous lump.

Attendance for screening to receipt of results	2 weeks
Receipt of result to attendance for assessment	2 weeks
Attendance for assessment to results of assessment	5 days
Attendance for assessment to open surgical biopsy	2 weeks
Final diagnosis to treatment	3 weeks

The actual wording of a standard is also important. Consider the following standard for a child care team: 'All children at risk will be investigated within one day'. This has several ambiguities which makes the standard difficult to monitor. For example, the team might not be informed that a child is at risk straight away – does the standard still apply? How do we define a child at risk? What do we mean by 'investigate' – is making one phone call sufficient? Does 'one day' mean the same day or 24 hours? Here is an alternative standard, which addresses these problems and is much more specific. Because it is more specific, it is easier to monitor and more likely to improve the quality of the service: 'All written or telephone referrals reporting that a child is at risk of physical or emotional abuse will be investigated within 24 hours of the referral being received. For each referral the area assessment form will be used and the plan of action agreed and signed by the duty senior'.

Hard and soft standards

Service standards should address both 'hard' and 'soft' dimensions. Hard standards are quantifiable – for example, the proportion of blood test results delivered to a GP within two working days, or answering 90 per cent of telephone calls within 15 seconds. Soft standards are qualitative – for example, being polite and courteous to customers.

The relationship between hard and soft standards can be illustrated by considering a rail company which wishes to monitor train delays. An example of a hard standard would be 'the proportion of trains arriving within ten minutes of the scheduled arrival time'. The problem with this standard is that although it is not difficult to measure, we do not know whether passengers would be satisfied with a delay of ten minutes and in any case this is likely to vary between different passengers who will have different views on whether a ten-minute waiting time is acceptable. Also it is a static measure. Even if there was an improvement in this standard, service quality could in fact be lower if, during the same period, expectations changed so that people were less willing to put up with a ten-minute delay.

There is another downside to using the 'hard' standard. It is well known that what gets measured affects behaviour. Anyone who has stood at a station looking at the arrivals screen for any length of time will have noticed that once a train starts to get behind schedule, the expected delay keeps increasing and increasing. My theory is that this is partly caused by the standards used. Once a train is, say, 20 minutes late and staff perceive that there is no way they can get the delay down to 10 minutes, there is a strong incentive for them to give priority to trains that are running less than 10 minutes late.

British Rail used to monitor delays of five minutes or more on inter-city trains. However, qualitative research indicated that passengers by and large were only dissatisfied if the train arrived more than ten minutes late. Of course, when British Rail changed the standard to ten minutes, people thought they were lowering their standards, but in fact they were trying to align their standards with what mattered to passengers.

'Satisfaction with the waiting time' is an example of a soft standard. It is about people's perceptions and experiences. Satisfaction is a more difficult concept to measure than delays. We could record the percentage of passengers who said that they were satisfied or very satisfied with the arrival time of trains, but this is only an indirect measure. Nevertheless, measuring the percentage of passengers who thought that any delays were acceptable does provide a much clearer link with customer satisfaction and will be of much use to the rail company.

Table 3.1 Examples of hard and soft standards

Hard standards	Soft standards
Decision on applications to adopt children within six months of formal application	Providing sensitive feedback to rejected applicants, stating clearly the criteria which have not been met
Number of inpatients waiting more than 15 months	Inpatients who thought that the waiting time was acceptable
Number of conceptions to girls under 16	Understanding and empathy shown to teenagers who are pregnant
Proportion of eligible 16- to 17-year-olds who are in care or care leavers having a pathway plan mapping out their route to independence	Practical support given to 16- to 17-year-olds who are in care or care leavers
Proportion of patients with coronary heart disease who have had a recorded blood pressure check in the last 15 months	Satisfaction with arrangements for obtaining prescribed medicine out of hours
Number of complaints relating to hospital and community geriatric services	Users with a disability satisfied that they were treated as a person

However, using soft standards without hard measures does lead to difficulties. First, it is only practical to get this information from a sample of passengers, and, despite modern survey techniques, the sample could be unrepresentative. Second, from the point of view of rail staff, the harder standard is easier to relate to and changes can be seen more easily.

Examples of hard and soft measures in health and social care are listed in Table 3.1. The above discussion on rail standards applies equally to monitoring inpatient waiting times. With the hard standard in the table, who is the admissions clerk likely to give preference to – someone who has been waiting 14 months, or someone who has been waiting 16 months? The examples of pathway plans and blood pressure checks given in Table 3.1 illustrate a point often made about hard standards. If these hard standards are met, users will not be dissatisfied, but they are unlikely to get particularly excited. Research indicates that hard standards are likely to lead to dissatisfaction if not achieved but will not necessarily give an organization a high rating if they are satisfactory. Soft standards on the other hand, if they succeed in making patients and service users feel special and treated as individuals, are more likely to make them very satisfied with their care.

Good practice in developing standards

When deciding what standards to adopt, it is important to consider both how they will improve the quality of service provided to service users and also what benefits they will have for staff. Many standards are rather vague and appear to be written primarily for public relations purposes. For standards to deliver service improvement they should be:

- *Realistic and attainable within available resources.* It is no good having standards that are beyond what can be achieved within resource constraints. This would only lower staff motivation and morale. If the standard that can be achieved is not what the customers require, then improvements will be needed in stages. One option would be to develop a standard that goes some way to meet those needs while informing users that this is just an interim standard and that efforts are being made to improve it.
- *Based on the views of service users.* The views of patients, carers and other service users can be obtained via a variety of feedback methods, both formal and informal, and will preferably result from direct discussion with patients and service users: 'users of services and carers must be involved in the identification and development of standards and in giving feedback to inform whether standards are met' (National Institute for Social Work 1999).
- *Real and important indicators of quality.* There is always a temptation to set standards that are easy to monitor but not necessarily central to the users' experience.
- *Expressed clearly and unambiguously.* It should be clear whether or not standards have been achieved.
- *Consistent with service aims and values.* They should take into account the views of managers, staff and other stakeholders. The organization must be able to demonstrate that it has a strategy to achieve its stated aims.
- *Set with the people who will be asked to achieve them.* If this does not occur, staff may be alienated by the standards rather than motivated by them. An important question when setting standards is who should participate in the process.
- *Measurable and capable of being monitored.* If they are not, then there will be no way to know to what extent they are being achieved. This is a controversial area, particularly in social care, as some social care standards are very difficult to measure.

The above characteristics are very useful in evaluating standards. In social care in particular, a wide range of national standards have been introduced in recent years. However, while there has been some representation from local authorities and the voluntary sector in developing the standards, many staff are angry that they have to meet measures that they feel are not realistic within existing resources and have not been set with the people who will be asked to achieve them. For example, the consultation document on fostering services (Department of Health 2001b) gives 195 minimum standards. While these standards appear to reflect service user views, it will be impossible for fostering managers and their teams – working mainly through volunteer foster carers – to ensure that they are all in place for all children in their care. Furthermore, the cost of monitoring all 195 standards would take away very valuable resources from the service itself.

Quality standards at Centrepoint

The service standards developed by Centrepoint illustrate the importance of taking into account both the immediate views of the young person and those of staff and managers. Centrepoint's original aim in 1969 was to ensure that no young person is at risk because they do not have a safe place to stay. This is still the same today. In order to develop its service standards, Centrepoint actively sought out the views of the young people using their services, and those of its staff, on what those standards should be. Examples of suggestions from the two different groups are given in Table 3.2.

It is clear that while the suggestions from staff and managers at Centrepoint have been developed with the young people in mind, they would not necessarily be raised by the young people themselves. Hence the importance of involving both parties. In some cases (e.g. regarding entertainment) young people's suggestions conflicted with Centrepoint's philosophy of helping users to become independent of the agency and be capable of using resources provided in the community. This was dealt with by making sure the young people understood this policy. However, it is important that Centrepoint do not dismiss the desire for entertainment. Either they should provide some

Table 3.2 Suggestions for standards at Centrepoint

Suggestions from young people	Suggestions from staff
Take away the uncertainty of having to move around to find a bed	Appeals procedure if young person feels discriminated against
Assistance with preparing for resettlement	Equal opportunities
Friendly staff	Empower young people and involve them
The building is clean, warm, comfortable and well-maintained	To take all allegations of harassment or abuse seriously
Safe place to live with secure building and equipment	Keep information about a young person confidential
Entertainment, outings and computers	Adequate notice of tenancy changes

Source: Casson and Johnson (1996).

limited form of entertainment or, and this will be preferable, make sure that the young people are welcomed at specific places in the community.

Quality standards at Capital Carers

A more comprehensive range of standards is given by Capital Carers, who aim to provide 'the full range of highest quality, best value care services which meet the personal social and health care needs of people wishing to remain at home' (Capital Carers 1998). They have a number of standards under the following headings: quality of life (for clients), quality of working life (for staff), quality of support, quality of management and quality of partnerships – see Table 3.3. These standards are viewed by Capital Carers as 'quality promises' which they make to their clients, carers, staff and purchasers. The process used to develop these standards had four phases: setting standards, monitoring them, evaluating outcomes and reviewing services.

Structure, process, outcome

Another issue for both social care and health is that *outcome* measures, whether quantified or not, may not measure the *process* of service delivery, and this may be crucial to quality. For example, staff may have developed a care plan within 48 hours of a user's referral, but has the user or carer contributed much to it? Has either had a chance to explore the options fully? Was the user given clear information about what will happen? Did the user and carer feel that their views were listened to?

Consider the difficulties in setting standards for the treatment of mental health patients. A standard could be set for certain client groups that they return to normal within so many months. But that would not be appropriate for most client groups. Even if it was, who is to say what is 'normal behaviour'? Who would monitor it – the person providing the service, the client or someone independent? Other examples include care of the elderly or of people with learning difficulties. Such areas require sophisticated standards that reflect some of the complexities of the service rather than simple counts of outcomes.

Donabedian (1980) addresses this problem by distinguishing between three critical components for written and measurable standards of care:

- *Structure*: the physical and organizational framework within which care is given. This includes the staff, facilities and equipment available, the environment within which the care is delivered and the documentation of procedures and policies.
- *Process*: the actual procedures and practices implemented by staff in their prescription, delivery and evaluation of care.
- *Outcome*: the effect of that care on the client, plus the costs of providing that care.

Table 3.3 Quality standards at capital carers

Quality of life	To provide a service tailored to the specific needs of clients and carers. To consult with clients and carers about what they want our service to achieve and on possible new services. To maintain and promote independence and the ability to stay at home as long as they wish. To maintain, and wherever possible, improve the quality of life for our clients and carers. To prevent a breakdown in care arrangements and avoid unnecessary admissions into hospital or residential care. To promote early discharge from hospital back home.
Quality of working life	Consult with staff regarding changes and developments. Provide appropriate management support, guidance and opportunities for personal development. Provide feedback on positive comments from their clients and carers. A quality of working life for staff which encourages them to develop their skills and maximize their own personal development. A working environment in which they feel supported and valued. A working environment which encourages them to remain with the organization. A genuine desire and commitment to providing the highest quality care to our clients and carers.
Quality of support	Continuity. Service provided regularly by a small team of community care workers that are known to them. A written care plan. Reliability. Worker will arrive within 15 minutes of a scheduled visit. To be informed by telephone, giving reasons, if the care worker will be late. Flexibility. We will respond appropriately to medical emergencies. That all requests for a varied service will be considered and met wherever possible. Attitudes of staff. To treat clients and carers with dignity and respect and relate to them in a kind and caring manner. Training. Care workers will have the necessary skills to provide a high standard of care and will undertake training. Information. Clients and carers will be given a written service information pack containing all relevant details about Capital Carers.

Table 3.3 (*continued*)

	Communication. Details of how to contact staff, both during and outside of office hours. All staff carry an ID badge.
Quality of management	Organizational strategy. An annual strategy review with clear implementation plans.
	Employment practices. Recruitment and selection procedures which promote good practice, equal opportunity and anti-discriminatory practice, as well as complying with employment legislation.
	Staff management, training and development. Full induction programme for all new staff, regular supervision from line manager, training and development.
	Operational practices. Compliance with Charities Act and other legislation. Quality assurance system.
	Financial management and administrative procedures. Sound financial management and administrative systems developed in line with the changing needs of the organization.
	Monitoring, evaluation and review. Robust monitoring systems, an annual quality audit for evaluating and reviewing services.
Quality of partnerships	Encouraging clients and carers to be involved in decisions relating to their care and the manner in which their care is provided. Taking all reasonable steps to protect clients and carers from abuse and exploitation.
	Supporting care staff if subjected to racist or sexist behaviour with the aim of finding a satisfactory resolution to the problem.
	Meeting service specifications and contract requirements of purchasers and funders. Work with purchasers and funders in identifying future needs and services.
	Discuss with relevant agencies any concerns regarding the quality of care being provided to particular clients.

Source: Capital Carers (1998).

This concept is well illustrated by a hair salon. The accommodation, equipment and training of staff are all part of the 'structure' element; the hairdressers' apparent skill and conversation are 'process' elements; while the appearance of the hair when the customer leaves is an 'outcome' element.

The importance of the three different components will vary depending on the nature of the service being offered. For people with learning difficulties

.

or in residential homes, the 'process' is often thought to be the most import-ant. Koch (1991) on the other hand believes that 'outcome is more difficult to define than structure and process standards and is arguably the most important of the three'. In fact, the three types of standard are interrelated. As Harr (2001) points out: 'only if we have a sufficient infrastructure will we be able to create stable, and therefore reproducible, processes. And only by having stable processes will we be able to achieve quality outcome'.

A problem with outcome measures in health and social care is that many outcome measures can only be evaluated after a long period of time. For example, a frequent outcome measure for patients with breast cancer is the five-year survival rate. While this is a vital indicator from the patient's view-point, by the time such measures are available, processes are likely to have changed and staff will have moved on. As Nicholls *et al.* (2001) point out, it is then too late to apply improvement initiatives based on the feedback.

Structure, process and outcome in community mental health

An example of the use of the structure, process and outcome headings for Somerset Health Authority's adult mental health service is given by Burbach and Quarry (1991):

- *Structure* refers to aspects of the physical environment (e.g. quality of decor and furnishings, accessibility of unit to clients) and to certain characteristics of the social environment (e.g. staffing ratios, skill mix). These are all relatively static factors or fixtures which generally do not change much during an episode of client contact.
- *Process* is concerned with events during a treatment episode. Typical process factors include nature and speed of response to referrals, allocation of cases, decisions about treatment to therapy, therapist time per client, and case-note recording.
- *Outcome* refers to the results of the team's intervention. It can be considered in terms of the extent to which the client has been helped or her/his problem resolved, and is a direct measure of the clinical effectiveness of treatment or therapy. Other outcomes might relate to the degree of client satisfaction with the service, or the extent to which the need for other specialised or costly services (e.g. acute psychiatric admissions), has been reduced.

Monitoring service standards

Developing service standards is a time-consuming process, but it can focus attention on problem areas and suggest immediate improvements. However, the main benefits come from sustained monitoring of performance against standards. If the service is not meeting the standard, there is work to be done

% seen within 30 minutes

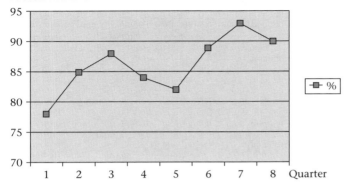

Figure 3.3 Monitoring the time taken to see patients

to find out the reasons and address the problems (preferably without search-ing for scapegoats). If performance is better than expected, the reasons should still be identified, so that ways may be found to continue to improve. As illustrated earlier in Figure 3.1, monitoring the service against the standards, identifying non-conformances and establishing their causes are all important ingredients in improving service quality.

The method chosen for monitoring depends to some extent on how the standards have been drawn up. Though many different factors may be meas-ured and compared, there are essentially four main approaches:

- record as a percentage the number of occasions when the standard is achieved;
- record whether the standard has been achieved, partially achieved, or not achieved in the period being considered;
- find out the degree of satisfaction of patients and service users with the performance on a particular standard;
- ask patients and service users whether they agree or disagree with a par-ticular statement.

An example of the first method is monitoring a standard to see a particular group of patients within 30 minutes of their arrival time. This is illustrated in Figure 3.3.

Some standards – for example the three standards from surgical nursing listed in Table 3.4 – cannot be measured in such a simple, quantitative way. The way forward in such cases could be to tick the appropriate column to indicate whether the standard was achieved, partially achieved or not achieved. The final column, though blank in this example, is perhaps the most crucial.

The third method of monitoring standards is to assess the degree of satis-faction of patients and service users with regard to a particular standard. This is discussed further in Chapter 9. Examples of some standards which are best

Table 3.4 Monitoring surgical nursing standards

Outcomes for good quality service	Achieved	Partially achieved	Not achieved	Further action to be taken
Regular clinical training	✓			
Care planned during the day to minimize disturbance to patients at night		✓		
Full and correct use of the nursing process documentation, with careful evaluation		✓		

Source: based on Koch (1991: 49).

Table 3.5 Monitoring satisfaction

	Very dissatisfied	Dissatisfied	Satisfied	Very satisfied
Friendliness of staff				
Explanation about what is happening to you				
Quality of meals				

monitored in this way are given in Table 3.5. Here, a four-point scale is used, but some people prefer a middle column, 'neither satisfied nor dissatisfied', as well.

The final approach is similar to the above in that it asks patients and service users to rate the service, but asks them whether they agree or disagree with a particular statement. Figure 3.4 shows an example used in Worcestershire County Council (Adams 1998).

There are, in turn, a number of ways in which an organization could collect the information it needs:

- ask staff to complete monitoring forms and correlate these centrally, perhaps using a computer;
- measure some standards, but otherwise expect staff to monitor their own practices;
- carry out spot checks on files;
- review cases with patients and service users present and check on the main standards;
- communicate standards to patients and service users and ask them to complain if they are not met;
- send patients and service users questionnaires to check on standards;

EXAMPLE STATEMENT

My social worker provided me with clear information about what services were available on leaving hospital and how to obtain them

Strongly								Strongly
disagree	1	2	3	4	5	6	7	agree

Figure 3.4 Measuring user perceptions
Source: Adams (1998).

- set up a group of staff, or 'quality circle', to monitor activity against standards and to plan improvements;
- invite someone from outside the department to review its work.

A combination of monitoring methods is usually necessary, and it can be a costly and complicated process. Beyond monitoring is the issue of intervention. Are there plans for improvement where standards are not being met? Has the problem been investigated? Are standards unrealistic? Are there targets to improve the service beyond the standards set?

Monitoring standards in child protection

Monitoring standards in child protection is not a straightforward task as there are many interested parties, some of whom might have been reluctant or angry about having to take part. However, even in this situation it is important to get the views of all participants. Table 3.6 gives examples of some standards for a child protection investigation and how they might be monitored using feedback from parents and carers. The actual feedback could be obtained either by asking them directly or by giving them a questionnaire.

Monitoring standards in contracts and partnership arrangements

There are a large number of partnership arrangements, contracts and service-level agreements in health and social care. These developments can offer the opportunity for greater flexibility and quality at lower cost, but for these benefits to be realized the commissioning organization needs to develop appropriate and cost-effective measures to ensure that contracted-out services are of high quality.

Table 3.6 Monitoring standards in child protection

Standard	Feedback from parents/carers
Parents will be informed about the different stages in a child protection investigation and their role in it.	Were you told about the stages in a child protection investigation, in a way you could understand? Did you understand the part you would play in the investigation?
Parents will not be judged as being guilty before the investigation.	Before the investigation, did you as parents/carers feel social workers judged you as being guilty of child abuse or not preventing it?
Case conferences will be of an appropriate size to gain relevant information about a case but without being intimidating to parents.	Did you feel the child protection conferences made it easy for you to make your point? Did you feel the people at these conferences listened to you? Were there any other professionals who you feel should have attended?
Staff will attend appointments made with parents/family within 30 minutes of the agreed time.	Did the social worker arrive within 30 minutes of the agreed time?
A written child protection plan is constructed with the involvement of the child, the child's parents/carers and relevant agencies.	After the child was placed on the Child Protection Register, did child protection staff listen to your ideas as parents/carers when writing the Child Protection Plan?

Source: based on Casson and Manning (1997: 44–5).

A key element of measuring performance in partnership arrangements and contracts is the development of the specification. Specifications tell the supplier or provider what is wanted and provide a basis for judging whether they have delivered this. They can also tell patients and service users precisely what they should expect from a service and so can serve as an important vehicle for empowering them. For staff, a specification clarifies what they are expected to do and how to do it. Introduced properly and collaboratively, a specification can also empower staff to take personal responsibility for achieving and improving standards.

Ideally, a specification should include the details needed to build up a precise picture of any services or goods that are being commissioned or provided. For example, describing a home for older people as a building in which a number of older people live and are looked after by a number of staff is a specification, but it gives only the barest information necessary. It is not sufficiently detailed to convey any impression of scale, lifestyle, quality of care or any of the other things a prospective resident would wish to know. Similarly, 'supply breakfast' may be all that a catering contract for an older people's home stipulates, but there are many other factors to consider even in this apparently simple requirement. On a practical level, details such as where and when breakfast should be served and what food is provided are left unresolved. On a qualitative level, the quality of food provided, how much choice residents are given and how far individual needs should be catered for are all left open to the provider's discretion. Such a wide brief is unsatisfactory both from the point of view of the purchaser, whose expectations of the service may be disappointed, and the provider, who may be frustrated by failing to provide a satisfactory service.

A specification for a service has to encompass the purpose and practical implications of the service, as well as the achievements and benefits expected of it. It needs to include sufficient detail to ensure effective communication, but not so much that it removes any possibility of sensible interpretation. The following pointers may prove helpful in drawing up a specification (Moullin 1999):

- Be as clear as possible about the outcomes that are wanted from the service – the vision.
- Recognize that the specification is part of a continuing process of improvement in the light of experience, and that the capacity for change and growth has therefore to be built into the design of a service.
- There are potentially a large number of interested parties, and a specification is the product of a negotiated process.
- Creativity and respect for others are crucial resources and working relationships need to foster them.
- It is ultimately the benefits to service users and patients that matter when evaluating a service. The original vision, representing a desire to achieve certain outcomes, has to be tested against actual outcomes.

Having drawn up a specification and established standards, the next stage in ensuring quality in contracts and service-level agreements concerns effective monitoring of standards. Without effective monitoring of quality, it is impossible to ensure that partnership arrangements are delivering a quality service. However, many commissioning authorities in health and social care have not developed the skills to monitor the quality and value for money of the services they have contracted out. In particular they do not always know what data to collect or how to interpret it. Also there can be a breakdown in the personal relationships and informal contact that form a vital part of monitoring.

The way in which the quality of services supplied to your enterprise or organization is monitored will partly be determined by the nature of the standards used in the specification. Where the service has been specified in terms of outcomes, monitoring will be based on observing and measuring them. The results will be compared with the standards or levels set out in the contract. Examples of outcomes include the impact of the service on patients and service users (e.g. a measurable improvement in their health and well-being). The quality of a service is often indivisible from the process through which the service is delivered, such as how the provider relates to service users and carers. Surveys, spot checks or continuous monitoring may then be needed. Another approach is to check that the contractor provides adequate inputs. For example, the number of staff used and whether they have the right skills and training. Measuring the outputs of the service is another possibility. The number of clients using the service and the number of patients treated are examples of output measures. Other measures which could be used are efficiency measures. These would include the cost of a service per client or per hour.

Arguably, outcome measures may be the most important. However, measurement is not easy. For example, in a project to educate young people about the dangers of drug use through outreach work, it is difficult to measure the increase in knowledge or whether this has resulted in a change in their behaviour. A survey of young people would provide some of this information, but useful measures include the number of people contacted (an output measure) and changes in levels of drug usage in the locality, compared with other areas.

For any service, a decision has to be made about the minimum number of performance indicators or standards to use. There should be enough indicators to provide a sufficient description of the service, yet not so many that an additional bureaucracy is necessary to collect the data. Many staff in voluntary organizations said that while they spent a lot of time and effort collecting the data they were asked for by local authorities, they were not sure that anyone actually looked at it (Bemrose and MacKeith 1996). It is also important to make sure that frequent meetings take place between the different organizations and that informal contacts do not disappear.

Consideration must also be given to the views of service users. As many ways as possible, both formal and informal, should be explored for involving service users and encouraging them to feel they have a contribution to make. Ultimately this will only succeed if staff do not feel threatened by this process. Though there is no one correct approach, because health and social care are provided for vulnerable and dependent people, trust and openness are of great importance.

Quality systems

It is relatively easy to pay lip-service to quality, trying to convince customers, employees and even oneself that the organization offers quality. However, to be sure of providing quality products and services consistently, the organization needs a *quality management system*. The Department of Health (1998a) agrees: 'Quality is not an add-on. It must be an integral part of coherent, consistently applied systems that continually involve the whole organisation in work to plan, deliver and evaluate the quality of services'.

For quality systems to work effectively, everyone needs to be involved and to understand what the organization is trying to achieve. One way to be sure that information is available to everyone is to write it down. Most organizations have manuals for individual procedures and people may feel resistant to adding to the paperwork. However, in such organizations, a quality management system or quality manual should actually reduce the bureaucracy rather than add to it. Some organizations will have several procedures for the same thing – for example, one had eight possible forms for filling in expense claims – while others have procedures which are either incomplete, long-winded or out of date.

If an organization has no procedures written down then the advantages of documenting the process of its work will be considerable. This will reduce confusion and improve quality because the process of writing up the procedures will lead to identification of what is best practice. In addition, it will make the training of new staff much easier.

Stebbing (1990) likens a quality management system to a life insurance policy. Provided payments are made regularly, the policy will protect the family against sudden bereavement. Similarly, a quality management system, if regularly monitored for effectiveness, will enable the company to keep going without losing momentum in the event of any changes in management or workforce.

A well-developed quality management system will indicate when and how any task is to be properly undertaken and by whom. It will also ensure that the organization meets and will continue to meet customer needs and expectations. I remember hearing on the radio a plea from a major brewery in the Midlands for one of its computer programmers who was on holiday 'somewhere in Scotland' to return as production had stopped because no one else knew how to modify one of their computer systems. In this case, the absence of a quality management system led to the loss of several days' production.

The basis of a quality management system, according to Oakland (2000), is illustrated in Figure 3.5. The starting point for a quality system is to write down what staff currently do. If there are different practices operated by different people this is an opportunity for them to learn from each other and develop an even better procedure. The next stage is to justify what the organization does, making sure it is consistent with the requirements of your customers and if possible with those of a good international standard such as ISO9000 (see p. 83). The next step is to do what is written. There are many cases where an excellent quality manual bears little relationship to what actually goes on in the organization. Keeping records is of course important and the process should be reviewed by all staff working in the area. Finally, it should not be seen as a one-off exercise. It should be used as a basis for continuing improvement and kept up to date.

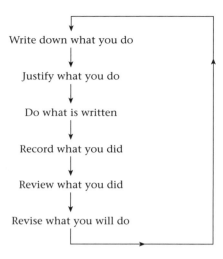

Figure 3.5 The quality system loop
Source: Oakland (2000).

The essence of a quality system is as follows:

- *a fully documented description* of the procedures used to provide the product and/or service, including a specification of the materials and equipment required;
- appropriate checks that the system is being *operated correctly and consistently* and without incurring unnecessary costs;
- appropriate checks to make sure that the service continues to *meet customers' requirements*.

A good approach to developing a quality system is to use the 12 headings given in the MQM2000 Public Sector standard designed by the Hull Quality Centre (Kingston upon Hull City Council 1999). In each of the 12 areas, an organization needs to develop procedures and to assemble some documentary evidence to show that each aspect has been covered appropriately. The 12 areas are:

- identifying key activities;
- controlling key activities;
- focusing on customer needs and expectations;
- understanding and meeting customer requirements;
- handling customer complaints;
- getting the best from your suppliers;
- looking after all materials and products;
- developing your people;
- keeping everyone informed;

- environmental management;
- measuring quality performance;
- making sure your quality system is working.

Quality systems in mental health

An example of a quality system in mental health services is the assessment pathway for older people with mental health problems developed by Wakefield and Pontefract Community and Mental Health NHS Trust. The Trust has developed a centralized assessment service with a single point of access and the assessment pathway was created to ensure that all users referred to older people's services receive the same standard of assessment. It is an evidence-based multi-professional pathway incorporating medical, nursing, occupational therapy and physiotherapy assessments, together with the older person's assessment of their own needs and problems and carers' perceptions of the person's difficulties. The pathway provides for an interim care plan within the first 24 hours following admission to an inpatient assessment unit (or the first visit) and a more detailed plan within 72 hours or three visits. In each case specific tasks and assessments are laid down which should be completed by the various professionals within that time period.

The main benefits of this quality system were identified as follows (Northern and Yorkshire NHS Modernisation Programme 2001):

- consistency of approach;
- ensuring a well coordinated plan of assessment for each individual;
- ensuring that key elements of the assessment plan are carried out within agreed time scales;
- enhanced multi-professional working with clear understanding of team roles and skills.

ISO9000

ISO9000 is an International Standard for quality systems that can be used by all organizations, whether in manufacturing or service sectors. It aims to build quality at every stage and sets out how to establish an effective quality system with appropriate documentation.

ISO9000 was first released in 1987 and revised in 1994 and again in 2000. One of the problems of the previous versions of the standard was that an organization could still conform to the standard but at the same time produce substandard products of a consistently poor quality. For example, a company manufacturing engines achieved the standard despite the fact that its engines were noisy and polluted the atmosphere. However, if some of the engines had not been noisy or polluting, the company would not have received the standard! This is confirmed by a survey carried out for Lloyd's

Register Quality Assurance Limited which asked 400 quality managers about the benefits of ISO accreditation under the previous scheme (Osman 1996). While the majority of respondents cited the marketing advantages of the standard, only 9 per cent of managers cited 'increased customer satisfaction' and just 4 per cent cited 'more quality awareness/improved quality'.

The latest revision to the ISO9000 standard is both more focused on the customer and less biased to manufacturing companies. It has also been simplified in that there is just one standard that all organizations have to meet rather than separate ones depending on the nature of the organization. This is ISO9001:2000. There are in addition two other main documents. ISO9000:2000 defines the concepts and what the various terms mean, while ISO9004:2000 provides guidance aimed at further improving an organization's quality performance, but is not intended for certification purposes.

ISO9001:2000 is based on eight quality management principles, as listed below (International Standards Organisation 2000). These terms are familiar from our earlier discussion of quality management and show clearly the link with quality management and TQM.

- customer focus;
- leadership;
- involvement of people;
- process approach;
- system approach to management;
- continual improvement;
- factual approach to decision making;
- mutually beneficial supplier relationships.

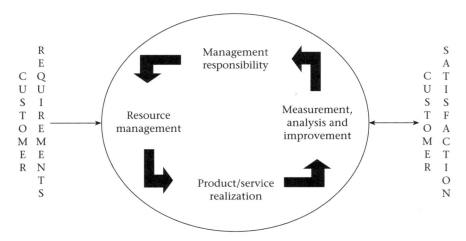

Quality management system

Figure 3.6   ISO9001:2000

The new model for ISO9001:2000 is illustrated in Figure 3.6. This shows clearly the cyclical relationship between the different aspects within the quality management system. It also shows the importance of customer requirements as a key input to the system and customer satisfaction as a key output.

Incidentally, to help in writing this section I rang the British Standards Institution Customer Services Desk to get information on the latest update to the ISO9000 standards. I got the following message: 'Our offices are now closed. Our office hours are Monday to Friday 8.30am to 5.30pm.' I looked at my watch and the time was 3.30pm on a Wednesday! An example of not practising what you preach!

Requirements of ISO9001

The organization's compliance with ISO9001 is evaluated in an initial assessment by the British Standards Institution. If successful, this is followed by regular unannounced surveillance visits to ensure that standards are maintained. As illustrated in Figure 3.6, to achieve ISO9001:2000 an organization has to satisfy the assessors in five areas:

- quality management system;
- management responsibility;
- resource management;
- product and/or service realization;
- measurement, analysis and improvement.

Within each of these five areas, an organization has to meet a number of requirements. These are listed below (based on International Standards Organisation 2000 and Praxiom 2001). The figures in brackets refer to the relevant subsections of the standard.

Quality management system

Develop and implement a quality management system, identifying key processes and describing them, and managing process performance (4.1).

Develop quality system documents, reflecting what the organization does, and prepare a quality system manual documenting procedures and how your processes interact. There also needs to be a control system to make sure all quality documents are kept up to date, ensuring only the most recent ones are used. You also need to maintain records to prove that the system is working effectively and requirements have been met (4.2).

Management responsibility

Promote the importance of quality and of meeting the requirements of customers and other stakeholders, including those required by law or by central government. Quality objectives must be set and there must be support from senior management for the quality system and sufficient resources must be provided. The quality management system must also be reviewed and improvements made accordingly (5.1).

Identify customer requirements, ensure that they are met and that customer satisfaction is enhanced (5.2).

Define your organization's quality policy and ensure it is aligned with corporate objectives and customer requirements. The quality policy should be widely communicated to people in the organization and reviewed regularly (5.3).

Formulate measurable quality objectives both for the organization as a whole and in functional areas. You also need to plan the development and implementation of the quality system and how it can be improved and modified (5.4).

There needs to be clearly defined responsibilities and authorities for quality, so that everyone knows their particular role in the system. These need to be communicated throughout the organization. Management's role also needs to be clear (5.5).

Review the quality system, evaluating its performance. Audit results, feedback from customers and process performance information all need to be monitored and corrective and preventive actions identified for any problems (5.6).

Resource management

Identify and provide the resources needed to support the quality system and to improve customer satisfaction (6.1).

Ensure that all staff have the right experience, education, training and skills. Identify and deliver training and awareness programmes (6.2).

Identify, provide and maintain buildings, workspaces, equipment, hardware and software, and support service needs (6.3).

Identify and manage the working environment to ensure services and products meet requirements (6.4).

Product and/or service realization

Plan and develop processes for producing products and services. Documents, quality control and record keeping systems also need to be in place (7.1).

Identify and review your customers' product and service requirements, including those imposed by external agencies. You must also ensure regular and effective communication with customers (7.2).

Plan and develop systems for product and service development, including inputs and outputs. Design and development reviews need to be carried out and changes in design need to be identified, recorded and validated (7.3).

Controls must be in place to ensure that purchased products and suppliers meet the specified requirements and appropriate documentation is kept (7.4).

Control and validate service activities, including processes, equipment, information and instructions given (7.5).

Ensure that all monitoring devices and controls are accurate (7.6).

Measurement, analysis and improvement

Plan and implement remedial processes when something goes wrong. Any problems must be systematically fed back to improve the process (8.1).

Measure customer satisfaction, products and processes, and perform regular audits (8.2).

Develop a procedure to control non-conforming products and correct them where possible. Records also need to be maintained (8.3).

Analyse data about your customers, suppliers, products and processes (8.4).

Use audits and other data about quality to generate improvements in the quality management system (8.5).

Benefits of ISO9000

ISO9000 has many benefits:

- it necessitates an explicit statement of declared aims or specifications;
- it requires a system for monitoring what the organization does and keeping records;
- it disciplines people to carry out audits and reviews of their systems;
- it helps people get to the root cause of problems;
- it ensures people define responsibilities fully;
- it gives a message that the organization is taking quality seriously: to patients, service users and partner organizations.

These advantages apply to health and social care as well as organizations in the public sector. A study by the British Quality Association (1990) concluded that 'ISO9000 offers a basis for managing social care and . . . benefit will be derived in terms of less wastage of time and effort due to poor organisation, with consequent advantages for those we seek to serve'.

ISO9000 at a residential home

Napier House is a local authority residential home in Newcastle, the majority of whose residents are elderly and mentally infirm. It was one of the first care organizations to become registered under ISO9000. The benefits of ISO9000 for residents included improvements in the treatment of incontinence which has ensured a greater level of hygiene and comfort, a greater voice in running their own home and in determining the treatment they receive, and a better complaints system. The benefits for staff included better documentation, particularly in the residents' files, which is not only uniform but simpler, more organized and easier to maintain. In medication, cross-checking ensures minimum risk to residents and their drug intake. Also, teamwork improved and 'staff gelled into an entity seeking a common purpose' (Humphrey and Hildrew 1992).

ISO9001 certification at a Swiss regional hospital

Staines (2000) identifies the following benefits of ISO9001 certification to a Swiss regional hospital:

- to force the organization to deal with both philosophical and operational quality issues;
- to accelerate the implementation of new legislation;
- to provide traceability;
- to bring a widespread feeling of pride and innovation;
- to ensure global re-examination;
- to ensure sustainable quality;
- to facilitate training of new staff members;
- to give staff members a more global understanding of their activities;
- to give staff members a comprehensive understanding of the hospital's activities;
- to provide a sound basis for, and an ambitious milestone on the way to, TQM;
- to demonstrate to the population the commitment towards TQM in the hospital.

However, Staines also found that ISO9001 did not deliver on the cultural dimension as it was fairly technical and formal. Things do not change in an organization because of new procedures, regulations and documentation. They change because people believe that they *should* change and *want* them to. This is done through a change in corporate culture, inspired and promoted by the management team. There should be a great impulse, a vision for a real quality spirit, prior to undertaking an ISO certification.

Guidelines for implementation

Gaining ISO9000 approval is a time-consuming task and one which needs to be properly planned. There are a number of ingredients for successful implementation. There needs to be evidence of commitment from senior management and the nominated coordinator must be seen to have authority. Adequate time needs to be set aside for the project and it should be seen as a continuous project without breaks and not delegated to someone to do in their spare time. There should be proper project management, planning who does what and when. Staff need to be involved in documenting procedures and to work as a team. In addition, good communication and feedback is required together with encouragement and recognition, and visible evidence of benefits.

Implementing ISO9000 for the Hertfordshire Home Care Service

Many people see ISO9000 as applying to private industry and manufacturing in particular. However, it can be applied successfully in both social care and health. One of the drivers for implementing the standard at Hertfordshire Home Care Service, one of the largest home care providers in the UK, was that it felt vulnerable to competition from the private sector. In addition to achieving ISO9002 (under the old classification) they received many other benefits. Costs of delivering the service fell by 14 per cent, home carer turnover fell by 10 per cent and the overall sickness rate for home carers fell by 25 per cent. There was increased continuity of care, with fewer home carers working with each client. This was achieved by creating teams of six carers. Due to greater flexibility, the home care service is now provided seven days a week. User satisfaction has risen. Finally, 'problems and issues are now looked at as an opportunity to refine the quality system, as opposed to blaming individual people' (Casson *et al.* 1997).

ISO9000 and the West Midlands Ambulance Service

When Paul Harris was appointed Market Development Officer for the West Midlands Ambulance Service (WMAS) after gaining ISO9000 certification for a Midlands steel manufacturer, he first thought that ISO9000 would not be at all appropriate in the ambulance service. However, he later talked about this to colleagues and they decided to investigate it further.

The big question was how to interpret ISO9000 for ambulance services. Communication was difficult because they were geographically and operationally fragmented and further complicated by the fact that they operated a shift system. It was impossible to call everyone together. The nearest organizations they could find who had looked at ISO9000 were in transport, but they quickly found that the differences far outweighed the similarities.

They took a number of steps before applying for ISO9000 certification:

- They talked in depth to other organizations with experience of ISO9000.
- They enlisted the help of management consultants who had experience of both quality systems and the health service.
- They appointed a quality assurance manager, John Williams, who was very well respected within the service.
- They set up a quality steering group, usually meeting once a week. This group also developed WMAS' quality policy: 'We will work together with our Customers and Suppliers both inside and outside the organisation to define and agree Quality Standards and Requirements. Our aim is to meet customers' requirements at all times. Our goal is continuous improvement in quality'.
- They set up a number of working groups to define and develop procedures for all activities of the service.

Table 3.7 Benefits of ISO9000 for WMAS

Staff	Managers	Organization
Standardized systems, consistent methods and procedures at all locations	Regular audits give feedback on performance	Improvement opportunities identified and followed up
Training in quality	Effective control of planned maintenance	Independent verification of good performance
Breaks with tradition	Encourages consistent performance	Produced saving in costs and time
Greater certainty: policy and expectations defined in writing	Improves communication	Helps meet changing needs
Builds commitment to the organization	Leads to a quality culture	

Documentation was a big problem. In fact it was observed that many of the procedures and practices already adopted by WMAS were consistent with ISO9000. However, this was not sufficient. They had to be written in a corporate style that was consistent with the needs of the whole of the service – a task which was not easy for some ambulance staff.

Once procedures had been written there were still problems in ensuring that staff both understood and accepted what was required. Establishing all aspects of quality beyond the care given to patients was to be a major task. To help the process they appointed a quality assurance coordinator, Alan Percival, to support the quality manager. Alan had previously been an operational ambulance man and could readily identify with and communicate with the main groups of staff. He was also able to explain the benefits that working to a quality system would bring.

Paul Harris listed the benefits of ISO9000 at WMAS for staff, managers and the organization as a whole (see Table 3.7).

WMAS have since used ISO9000 as the foundation for their approach to total quality. Building on the requirements of the standard, internal service level agreements have been established between all departments and regular assessments take place to measure improvements in performance. Its commitment to using a quality management system to best effect has been a major factor in diversifying its activities to include communications, health information and advice services. Barry Johns, Chief Executive of WMAS, concludes (Taylor 2001):

Our well-established ISO9001 quality management system has provided the bedrock for delivering our services . . . It has helped us to achieve an organisational philosophy and culture which encourages innovation, belief in its capabilities and the commitment to ensure that agreed targets are met.

Paul Harris offers this advice to people considering ISO9000:

- go for it but be realistic about what is involved;
- define what you want to achieve and how to do it;
- understand what is required;
- sell the benefits it is going to give you;
- bring staff and customers along with you;
- in the long term, going for quality service-wide is best rather than in one area, but do it on a scale you feel comfortable with.

ISO9000 and TQM

An organization that wishes to embark on a major quality improvement programme must decide whether ISO9000 is appropriate for its needs. If so, it needs to decide whether to go for the Standard first before embarking on a TQM-based approach, or to go for the Standard as part of a quality management programme. The main differences between the two approaches are summarized in Table 3.8. Tito Conti (1997) vice-president of the International Academy for Quality, summarizes the differences as follows: 'TQM models put emphasis on leadership, empowerment, delegation and debureaucratisation

Table 3.8 Comparison of ISO9000 and TQM

ISO9000	TQM
Focus on standards to ensure things are done right	Focus on doing things right and doing the right things
Primarily focused on products and services	Organization-wide
It is a system	It is a philosophy and an approach to management
No particular requirement for employee involvement	Emphasis on total employee involvement and commitment
Responsibility tends to lie with quality department	Emphasis on making everyone responsible
The goal is to meet the Standard and pass the audit	The goal is continuous improvement
Lower visibility	Organization-wide visibility

and teamwork, while ISO9000 was more focused on rigid standardisation of work processes, on procedures and on personal and functional responsibilities. The two were somehow on a collision course'.

Assuming the organization decides ISO9000 is appropriate, the best policy is to go for it as part of a quality management or continuous improvement initiative. However, it is tempting, particularly for smaller organizations, to conserve time and energy and go for the Standard first – and get external accreditation. The danger is that it may never get round to the quality management part.

Another potential problem of ISO9000 is that it was designed for static technologies and keeping it up to date in a rapidly changing world is a major problem. Hans Barajia, President of Multiface Inc. in Detroit, asks 'With the current rate of change, how can we find time to document the processes when what you want to do changes so often?'

Let us leave the last word to the American Society for Quality Control (ASQC). When comparing ISO9000 with the Baldrige Award and the Deming Prize, the ASQC states:

> You can't hope to meet the expectations of any of these programs if you aren't already implementing the ISO9000 standards in your company. These standards provide the foundation on which you can build your quality management and quality assurance systems so you may ultimately achieve a high level of success. Moreover, the ISO9000 series is the only system accepted internationally.
>
> (Quoted in Ross 1994)

PART two

Excellence

CHAPTER four

The Excellence Model

The Excellence Model was launched in 1991 by the European Foundation for Quality Management (EFQM), an organization formed in 1988 by 14 chief executives of leading European companies. The model was designed to enable organizations to assess themselves against a set of criteria for excellence and to use this self-assessment to identify and implement breakthrough improvements. The model also provides a framework for the European and UK Quality Awards, but the main aim is to stimulate quality improvement throughout Europe.

The model has been developed both for the public and private sectors. Originally known as the Business Excellence Model, it was redesigned in 1999 and the main reason that the model changed its name to the Excellence Model was to make it clear that it applied to *all* organizations. In the UK public sector it has been applied to local authorities, health and social care, schools, universities, all the police forces, the fire service, most central government departments and many voluntary sector organizations. There has been a Public Sector Award since 1995 and the model is particularly relevant to the modernizing agenda in public services. The model has received praise from many areas of health and social care.

What is excellence?

> We are what we repeatedly do. Excellence then is not an act but a habit.
>
> (Aristotle)

Before discussing the model in detail, it is useful to examine exactly what we mean by the term 'excellence'. In fact, excellence as a term suffers from many of the ambiguities associated with the word 'quality'. Perhaps this is not surprising since 'quality' is defined in Webster's dictionary and the Oxford dictionary as 'the degree of excellence'! In particular, does it mean technical excellence, excellence in a transcendent sense like a Rolls-Royce (see Chapter 1), excellence as the customer sees it, excellence in managing staff or excellence in keeping costs under control? In fact, excellence is all of these things, and we can say that: 'Organizational excellence is outstanding practice in managing organizations and delivering value for customers and other stakeholders'.

Basically, then, 'excellence' means excellence in everything! While it has many similarities to the term 'quality', its scope is wider. Whereas quality tends to be defined in terms of outcomes (e.g. customer satisfaction), excellence also includes process factors and additional results outcomes including financial and society results.

The EFQM Excellence Model

The basis of the Excellence Model is that excellence in the core service (be it clinical excellence or care), customer satisfaction, financial performance, employee motivation and good corporate citizenship are just different aspects of an excellent organization rather than conflicting demands. In the words of the EFQM, 'Excellent results with respect to Performance, Customers, People and Society are achieved through Leadership driving Policy and Strategy, People, Partnerships and Resources, and Processes' (EFQM 1999).

The model has nine elements each of which is used to assess an organization's progress towards excellence (see Figure 4.1). The first five are *enablers*, which are concerned with *how* results are being achieved, and the other four are *results* concerned with *what* is achieved.

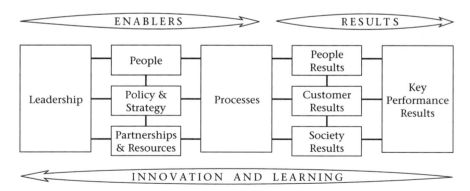

Figure 4.1 The Excellence Model
Source: EFQM (1999). © EFQM. The EFQM Excellence Model is a registered trademark.

In using the model an organization will typically start by examining the results categories: what are the key performance results that matter most for the organization or department, what are the main results from the point of view of staff and customers, and what matters to those in society who are not direct service users? Then the team using the model will evaluate how well they are doing based on these performance criteria and identify areas for improvement. Typically, while an organization will have some measures for many of these aspects, for others they will have none and part of the task will be identifying new and more relevant measures of performance.

Once the results have been analysed, the next stage is to identify the strategy for improving performance against the relevant criteria – and this is where the enablers come into play. If, for example, self-assessment of the results elements indicate that service users are not happy with a particular part of the service, then the real reason for this could be lack of leadership, it could be poor people management, it could be that the policies and strategies are not focused on the customer, it could be a failure in partnership working with other agencies or in managing resources, or it could be that the processes are poorly designed. Most likely it will be a combination of two or three enablers that need to be put right.

The model aims to avoid simplistic solutions. For example, if staff feedback (part of people results) is not very positive, it is tempting to put the blame on poor people management. However, it could just as easily be caused by poor leadership, poor processes putting strain on staff, lack of support from other agencies, inadequate resources or unclear policies and strategies. The model provides a framework for identifying where improvements need to be made.

Finally, do not ignore the innovation and learning dimension. The model can be used to improve things little by little, but is also ideally suited for helping staff identify breakthrough solutions where doing things differently (some would use the word 'smarter') can make dramatic improvements. Also, much can be achieved by learning from, and sharing best practice with, other organizations.

According to Pavlou and Chisnell (1997) the benefits from using the model at Salford Royal Hospitals NHS Trust included the following:

- providing a common language for a comprehensive performance management system which is readily acceptable to clinical and non-clinical staff alike;
- providing a common framework for measuring, focusing on and improving key results in all parts of the organization;
- putting quality improvement initiatives at the heart of day-to-day operational activity;
- being enthusiastically welcomed by staff involved as a powerful means of communicating their pride or concerns about the way the organization is operating and developing;

- providing the opportunity to involve all staff in the setting of priorities;
- enabling the Trust to benchmark against others in the NHS and outside;
- providing a basis for measuring health care excellence which is sensitive to local circumstances and professional priorities.

Underlying concepts of the Excellence Model

The underlying concepts of the Excellence Model are illustrated in Figure 4.2. At the heart of the model is *customer focus*, concentrating on the requirements and expectations of customers. For health and social care, the appropriate phrase is 'patient and service user focus'. The word 'carer' should also be in there, but is omitted to keep the phrase short.

In some ways this is just stating the obvious as it is the fundamental purpose of the service. However, in thousands of decisions day in and day out within health and social care, the interests of service users (patients and carers) are not in fact at the forefront. The convenience of staff and adherence to procedures designed without any involvement of patients or carers often relegates the needs of users to second or third place.

In many health services there has been a reluctance to publicly acknowledge this focus – indeed, many managers still talk about 'meeting the needs of staff and service users' and are resistant to changing the order to 'service users and staff'. While the needs of staff are important, the service exists for the users and needs to be designed around them. Of course it is impossible to provide a good service if the needs of staff are not met, but the needs of the service user and patient must come first.

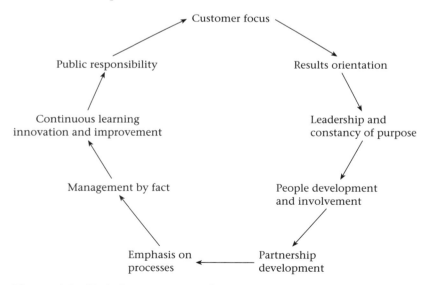

Figure 4.2 Underlying concepts of the Excellence Model

Leadership and constancy of purpose is also fundamental to the model. Constancy of purpose is the phrase of W. Edwards Deming (see Chapter 2). It refers to a long-term commitment by the senior management team and chief executive to quality improvement. It means that an initiative on quality will not disappear because of changes in personnel, a short-term funding crisis or other pressures. This commitment underpins all the work on quality.

People development is another underpinning factor. Excellence for patients and service users is only obtained through the large numbers of staff working in health and public services. People development involves training and developing staff both in their core professional roles and in the culture of customer focus, team working and supporting staff in providing services for service users. It requires openness, the ability to listen to colleagues and users, the recognition that communication and partnership working are the key and that a blame culture – putting the blame on individuals, other staff groups and even users – for poor service is counter-productive.

In addition to developing people, *people involvement* is also vital. There are two main reasons for this. First, a large number of staff towards the bottom of the hierarchy are in daily contact with users. They will know the needs of particular users better than many managers and will have a variety of ideas for improving the service, based on both users' views and experiences and their own. Tapping into this rich resource is very important indeed. Second, if staff are alienated and do not feel valued by their managers or by other professionals they will not be providing the best service they can. Involving staff in decisions affecting the service they provide is very important to get their goodwill and to make them feel valued. Empowerment of staff – in particular developing staff and giving them the authority to make decisions within a given framework without reference to senior colleagues – is another aspect of people involvement.

Partnership development is an area talked about a lot throughout the public sector, but examples of real partnership working are less common. A high proportion of service users have needs which transcend individual services. In a hospital patients will see a variety of staff in one visit – reception, X-ray, physiotherapy, catering etc. – while many service users will be attended to by a variety of professionals. In order to provide a seamless service, staff in the various departments need to work closely together. Partnerships between health and social care are also important whether in hospital discharge, child protection, alcohol and other drug misuse or mental health.

An emphasis on looking at *processes* is another vital aspect of the Excellence Model. We all have processes – whether for admitting patients to hospital, ordering medical supplies, allocating work to staff, assessing potential foster carers or providing meals in a residential home. Many of these processes will have been the same for years. They may not be written down – just based on custom and practice – and the reason for some of the stages in a process may have long been forgotten. In particular they may be over-complicated or miss out a key stage vital for a quality service. In some cases processes are written down but there are several different versions in circulation and it is not clear which is current. Writing down and re-examining processes with staff and users, cutting out any unnecessary stages, is a key method for improving the service.

Management by fact is another fundamental concept of the EFQM Excellence Model. It means not just relying on hearsay, but systematically collecting information about relevant factors and performance measures and using that information to redesign processes to provide better quality services. While 'the NHS culture is not – by and large – one which encourages reporting and analysis' (Department of Health 2000a) this is an area which is beginning to be addressed within health and social care. The increasing emphasis on evidence-based practice and the National Institute for Clinical Excellence (NICE) are examples of this. Both of these aim to ensure that decisions are based on facts, not just on staff opinions.

Continuous learning is another underlying concept. It means that we analyse results and the performance of an organization and use this information to improve processes. As with management by fact, there is room for improvement within health and social care: 'In general, the NHS does not appear to learn lessons consistently or quickly from the systems that are currently available to it, though there is some good practice on which to build' (Department of Health 2000a). The RADAR concept discussed later in this chapter is an example of this, as is the Deming cycle (see Chapter 2).

Innovation and improvement refers to the essentially radical nature of the Excellence Model. When evaluating a service, it is important to stand back and see if a process can be radically changed through some, usually fairly simple, innovation or change. Innovation and improvement is about challenging services, as with Best Value, and asking fundamental questions: why do we provide this service and how else could we achieve our objectives? An organization should also look at others, both in the same sector and elsewhere, to see how they perform similar activities.

The notion of *public responsibility* is very relevant to health and social care and other public organizations. They need not only to satisfy their patients and service users, but also to be a responsible employer that cares for its staff and the environment. They also need to demonstrate that their values are consistent with society's expectations – for example, on equity and access to services.

The final basic concept of the model is that of *results orientation*. This recognizes that excellence is about satisfying the needs of all relevant stakeholders – staff, service users, partners, government and society in general. Good performance on the enablers without delivering results for the key stakeholders is not sufficient.

The Excellence Model and TQM

A frequently asked question is how does the use of the Excellence Model compare with TQM. Specifically, is it just another approach to achieve the same end or does it represent something different?

While the Excellence Model is based on TQM – indeed, it was designed by the EFQM – it is more ambitious in scope. In private industry for example, profitability is not explicitly mentioned in TQM, but will be a key performance result in the Excellence Model. Tim Melville-Ross, Director General of the Institute of Directors, explains the difference between the two quite well: 'The EFQM Excellence Model is more than just a framework for quality. It is also a way of achieving excellence in the round: excellence in the way that an organisation manifests itself to its employees, shareholders and neighbours' (Institute of Directors 1997).

Death by 100 initiatives

Another frequent question is whether the Excellence Model is just the latest in a line of initiatives that organizations have to deal with. What with ISO9000, IiP, TQM, the NHS Plan, Best Value, Quality Protects and Clinical Governance, some managers ask whether this isn't at least one initiative too many.

Mike Perides (formerly Public, Voluntary and Health Sector Manager for the British Quality Foundation) gives the example of a woman who goes to a bar and orders three pints of beer, two gin and tonics and a tomato juice. The barman asks, 'Do you want a tray for that?' and she replies, 'Can't you see, I've got enough to carry already.' The Excellence Model, Perides continues, is like the tray: other initiatives can fit into one or more of its nine boxes. It can provide an overall framework enabling people to see the relationships between different initiatives while identifying the benefits in terms of results. It also makes clear to staff that all their work on other initiatives is not wasted, and that the Excellence Model is not just the next one, soon to be abandoned when the next collection of buzzwords comes in.

As an example, the Inland Revenue Accounts Office in Cumbernauld, which won the European Quality Award in 2000, had used a variety of quality-related schemes for a number of years. These included employee involvement (see Chapter 6), customer awareness workshops, IiP and Charter Mark. The problem was that while solutions were working successfully on an individual basis, they were working in isolation. By using the model, previously separate initiatives were joined into one practical framework.

Another example is St Mungo's, the largest homelessness charity in London. They had worked previously with both IiP and ISO9000. Kate Lattimore, Quality and Policy Coordinator at St Mungo's, says that 'one of the attractions of the Model is that it provides a framework that can incorporate both of the other quality standards on which we have been working . . . Our work using the Model is a continuation of our existing quality work, rather than being a separate and distinct initiative' (Quality Standards Task Group 2001).

Table 4.1 shows the main links between various quality-related initiatives and the different elements of the model. If an organization has worked with IiP, for example, this can be fed into the work on the model, particularly

Table 4.1 The relationship between different quality initiatives

Element	IiP	ISO9000	Clinical Governance	Best Value	Charter Mark
Leadership	*				
Policy and strategy		*	**		
People management	**				
Partnerships and resources				**	
Processes		**	**	*	
People results	**				
Customer results		*	*	*	**
Society results					
Key performance results		*	**	**	**

Key: ** a strong link; * quite a strong link. If blank, then a weaker link or none at all.

under people management and people results. Note that the ISO9000 column is based on the previous version of the standard, as there is little evidence as yet from the more recent ISO9000:2000.

For organizations using Best Value, the model provides an integrative framework which is not present in Best Value and again shows clearly how other aspects (e.g. leadership and people management) are needed for Best Value to be effective. As mentioned in Chapter 2, many local authorities and services are using the Excellence Model alongside Best Value.

The Excellence Model has also proved useful for Clinical Governance. What the model provides is a framework showing the relationship between clinical and non-clinical services in delivering care to patients. As Henry Stahr, Excellence Development Manager at Salford Royal Hospitals NHS Trust, says: 'For clinical care to flourish the whole organization, clinical and non-clinical, have to focus together on the needs of the patient and work together in an integrated way'.

In order to deliver the results required for Clinical Governance, all the enablers are relevant, as are each of the four results categories. Wakefield and Pontefract Community Health NHS Trust have used the model as a framework for the comprehensive mapping of the elements that need to be in place to deliver Clinical Governance. This is illustrated in Figure 4.3.

Model criteria and sub-criteria

Each element of the Excellence Model is broken down into a number of parts or sub-criteria. Specifically for each sub-criterion, the assessment team needs to identify the organization's strengths and areas for improvement. Definitions of the nine elements, together with the sub-criteria for each are shown in Table 4.2.

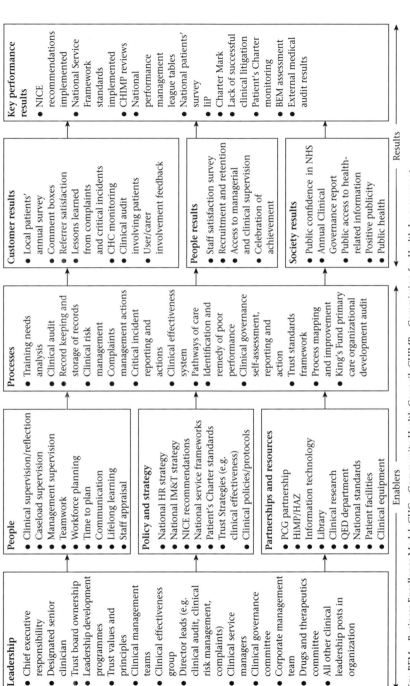

Key: BEM = Business Excellence Model; CHC = Community Health Council; CHIMP = Commission for Health Improvement; HiMP/HAZ = Health Improvement/Health Action Zone; IM&T = information management and technology; HR = human resources; IM&T = information management and technology; PCG = Primary Care Group

Figure 4.3 Model of Clinical Governance in Wakefield and Pontefract Community Health NHS Trust

Table 4.2 Definitions and sub-criteria for the elements of the Excellence Model

Element	Sub-criteria
Leadership: how leaders develop and facilitate the achievement of the mission and vision, develop values required for long-term success and implement these via appropriate actions and behaviours, and how they are personally involved in ensuring that the organization's management system is developed and implemented.	Leaders develop the mission, vision and values and are role models of a culture of excellence. Leaders are personally involved in ensuring the organization's management system is developed, implemented and continuously improved. Leaders are involved with customers, partners and representatives of society. Leaders motivate, support and recognize the organization's people.
Policy and strategy: how the organization implements its mission and vision via a clear stakeholder-focused strategy, supported by relevant policies, plans, objectives, targets and processes.	Policy and strategy are based on the present and future needs and expectations of stakeholders. Policy and strategy are based on information from performance measurement, research, learning and creativity related activities. Policy and strategy are developed, reviewed and updated. Policy and strategy are deployed through a framework of key processes. Policy and strategy are communicated and implemented.
People: how the organization manages, develops and releases the knowledge and full potential of its people at an individual, team-based and organization-wide level, and plans these activities in order to support its policy and strategy and the effective operation of its processes.	People resources are planned, managed and improved. People's knowledge and competencies are identified, developed and sustained. People are involved and empowered. People and the organization have a dialogue. People are rewarded, recognized and cared for.
Partnerships and resources: how the organization plans and manages its external partnerships and internal resources in order to support its policy and strategy and the effective operation of its processes.	External partnerships are managed. Finances are managed. Buildings, equipment and materials are managed. Technology is managed. Information and knowledge are managed.
Processes: how the organization designs, manages and improves its processes in order to support its policy and strategy and fully satisfy (and generate increasing value for) its customers and other stakeholders.	Processes are systematically designed and managed. Processes are improved, as needed, using innovation in order to fully satisfy and generate increasing value for customers and other stakeholders.

Table 4.2 (*continued*)

Element	Sub-criteria
	Products and services are designed and developed based on the needs and expectations of customers and other stakeholders. Products and services are produced, delivered and serviced. Customer relationships are managed and enhanced.
Customer results: what the organization is achieving in relation to its external customers.	Perception measures. The perceptions of service users and other stakeholders of the organization's image, services, support, and on their loyalty to the organization. Performance indicators. Internal indicators also relating to image, services provided, support and loyalty.
People results: what the organization is achieving in relation to its people.	Perception measures. People's perceptions of the organization. These include their motivation and job satisfaction. Performance indicators. Internal indicators relating to people's achievements, motivation, involvement and satisfaction, and also relating to the services provided to the organization's people.
Society results: what the organization is achieving in relation to local, national and international society as appropriate.	Perception measures. Society's perceptions of the organization on whether it has behaved responsibly, its involvement in the community, its environmental policies etc. Performance indicators. Internal indicators on the factors listed in 'Perception measures', together with others such as press coverage.
Key performance results: what the organization is achieving in relation to its planned performance.	Key performance outcomes. These are the key results planned by the organization and include financial and non-financial outcomes. Key performance indicators. These are the operational indicators and include those relating to processes, external resources (including partnerships and suppliers), financial, buildings, equipment and materials, technology and information and knowledge.

Source: EFQM (1999). © EFQM. The EFQM Excellence Model is a registered trademark.

Most of the terms used in Table 4.2 will be clear for public sector organizations. The differences between perceptions measures (which must come directly from staff, service users or people in society) and performance indicators (which can be collected internally) are described in more detail in Chapter 9. The term 'external customer' refers to the beneficiaries of the organization's activities, but may include other customers in the chain. For example, those of an acute hospital might include patients, carers, GPs and medical insurers, while those of a social services department might include children in need, carers, older people and other beneficiaries, and voluntary organizations.

Some public sector organizations find the society results criterion problematic. Surely, impact on society is the main aim of public sector organizations? To help resolve this it is useful to see why this criterion was introduced for business organizations. This was essentially to lodge the image of the organization with people who were not necessarily customers. Shell, for example, found that its attitude to the environment as perceived by the public needed to be monitored, as if its environmental policies were unacceptable its image and profitability would be adversely affected. In the public sector 'reputation in the community' might be a more useful way of looking at this. For example, a householder who has not been involved in crime, either as victim, witness or perpetrator, will nevertheless have a perception of the effectiveness of the police force. Also, members of the public will be concerned that children are protected from significant harm, while people who have been fortunate enough not to need any medical care in recent years will still be concerned about their nearby hospital. One of the difficulties in health and social care is that people's perceptions are influenced by the media. An organization's reputation in the community is also influenced by whether it appears to have behaved responsibly – for example, in relation to equal opportunities – by its involvement in the community and by its environmental policies.

Self-assessment using the Excellence Model

One of the Excellence Model's main purposes is self-assessment. Self-assessment has been defined as a 'regular, comprehensive and systematic review of an organisation's activities and results against a tangible and relevant model which culminates in the identification of the organisation's strengths and areas for improvement which facilitates the development and prioritisation of planned improvement actions' (Shergold and Reed 1996). Self-assessment using the model provides a rigorous and structured approach to business improvement, ensures an assessment based on fact and not opinion and enables the organization to achieve a consistency of direction and consensus on what needs to be done.

Self-assessment also enables organizations in health and social care to measure success and give improvement targets, to highlight and share best practices, to make comparisons between different areas or units, to create a vision or role model of excellence and to meet the requirements of patients, carers and service users more effectively:

> The self-assessment process offers the organisation an opportunity to learn. To learn about the organisation's strengths and areas for improvement. To learn about what TQM means when applied to your organisation. To learn about how far down the Quality road the organisation has travelled, how much further the organisation has to travel and how it compares with others.
>
> (Cabinet Office 1999)

Self-assessment can be carried out at the unit or department level and is best performed by a self-assessment team drawn from a broad cross-section of the functional areas, possibly with the help of external facilitators or trained assessors. The real usefulness of self-assessment will depend on how the areas identified for improvement are dealt with. If these are brushed under the carpet, or ignored, or dealt with in a piecemeal fashion, then the real benefits will not be obtained.

Using RADAR

The RADAR logic is an integral part of self-assessment using the Excellence Model. It consists of four elements: results, approach, deployment, assessment and review (see Figure 4.4). The logic states that an organization needs to:

- Determine the *results* it is aiming for as part of its policy and strategy-making process. These results cover the performance of the organization, both financially and operationally, and the perceptions of its stakeholders.

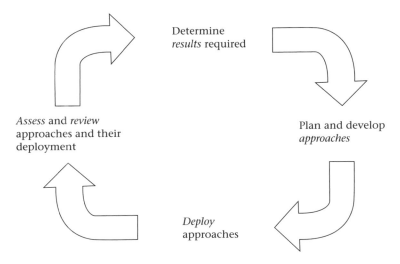

Determine
results required

Assess and *review*
approaches and their
deployment

Plan and develop
approaches

Deploy
approaches

Figure 4.4 RADAR

- Plan and develop an integrated set of sound *approaches* to deliver the required results both now and in the future.
- *Deploy* the approaches in a systematic way to ensure full implementation.
- *Assess* and *review* the approaches followed based on monitoring and analysis of the results achieved and on ongoing learning activities. Based on this, identify, prioritize, plan and implement improvements where needed.

As Kate Lattimore, Quality and Policy Coordinator at St Mungo's says, 'the RADAR logic has been a very useful and simple tool. We have tried using it in all our approaches as it requires that we first try to determine the results we are looking for, then plan what we have to do to meet these results and finally, assess and review to see if the results were achieved' (Quality Standards Task Group 2001).

When using the model within an organization, for example for the purposes of self-assessment, the approach, deployment, assessment and review elements of the RADAR logic should be addressed for each enabler sub-criterion, while the results element should be addressed for each results sub-criterion.

Scoring and self-assessment

So far in this chapter there has been no mention of scoring – giving scores for the organization or unit on each of the elements and sub-criteria. This is deliberate as scoring is not essential in the use of the model for continuous improvement. However, for self-assessment and benchmarking against other organizations or units, scoring has an important part to play.

The EFQM Excellence Model provides suggested weightings for each of the nine criteria, based on feedback from a wide consultation exercise across Europe. These are shown in Figure 4.5. While each organization is free to provide their own weightings which they feel are more appropriate to them, there are advantages for benchmarking purposes of keeping to the weights given. The percentage values shown are those used for the European and UK Quality Awards in developing an overall score for an organization. As can be seen the enablers and results categories carry equal weights of 50 per cent each. The figure also shows that the size of the boxes does not represent their importance – customer results having the highest individual weighting.

There are two main stages in self-assessment using the model: collecting all the information together, and then scoring the organization on the different criteria and sub-criteria. As with any scoring mechanism, however, there are possible pitfalls. If people score themselves, for example, it is difficult to ignore the fact that the score they give will affect other people's perceptions of how good they are and how their department is perceived relative to other departments. Some organizations (e.g. Lloyds/TSB) are considering not using scoring at all for this reason alone. Also there is a major difference between self-assessment using the model and applying for an award (e.g. the UK Quality Award). In the latter the emphasis is typically on making the assessor aware

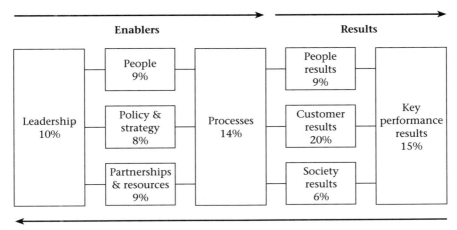

Figure 4.5   The EFQM Excellence Model showing criteria weightings
Source: EFQM (1999). © EFQM. The EFQM Excellence Model is a registered trademark.

of the organization's strengths, while minimizing the impact of the areas for improvement. In self-assessment the emphasis of these should be reversed.

The RADAR logic is used to score both enablers and results. The first R (results) relates to the scoring of results elements, while the other four elements of the logic (approach, deployment, assessment and review) relate to the scoring of enablers.

Scoring results elements

In developing a score for each results criteria, the sub-criteria for people results and customer results are weighted: perception measures 75 per cent and performance indicators 25 per cent. The weights for society results are perception measures 25 per cent and performance indicators 75 per cent, while those for key performance results are key performance outcomes 50 per cent and key performance indicators 50 per cent.

Five attributes are used in scoring each results sub-criterion, as can be seen from the sample scoring sheet in Figure 4.6. These are:

- Trends – are they positive, showing sustained good performance?
- Targets – have they been achieved and are they appropriate?
- Comparisons – have results been compared with other units or 'best in class', and if so how well do they compare?
- Causes – has the link between the approach taken and the particular results element been established?
- Scope – do the results measured address all relevant areas?

Attribute	A	B	C	D	E
Trends: Positive trends and/or sustained good performance	No evidence or anecdotal information	Positive trends and/or satisfactory performance on some results	Positive trends and/or sustained good performance on many results over at least 3 years	Strongly positive trends and/or sustained excellent performance on most results over at least 3 years	Strongly positive trends and/or sustained excellent performance on most results over at least 3 years
Targets: Targets appropriate and achieved	No evidence or anecdotal information	Favourable and appropriate in some areas	Favourable and appropriate in many areas	Favourable and appropriate in most areas	Excellent and appropriate in most areas
Comparisons: Comparisons indicate that results compare well with external organisations	No evidence or anecdotal information	Comparisons in some areas	Favourable in some areas	Favourable in many areas	Excellent in most areas and 'best in class' in many areas
Causes: Results are caused by approach	No evidence or anecdotal information	Some results	Many results	Most results	All results. Leading position will be maintained
Scope: Results address relevant areas	No evidence or anecdotal information	Some areas addressed	Many areas addressed	Most areas addressed	All areas addressed

Figure 4.6 Scoring results with the EFQM Excellence Model
Source: Based on EFQM (1999). © EFQM. The EFQM Excellence Model is a registered trademark.

The process of scoring each attribute is to tick the most appropriate statement in each row. Typically column A equates to with a score of 0 per cent for that attribute, column B 25 per cent, column C 50 per cent, column D 75 per cent and column E 100 per cent. An overall total is then given for each element based on the scores for each attribute.

Scoring enablers

There are three steps to scoring enablers using the Excellence Model. These are shown in the scoring sheet for enablers in Figure 4.7. The first step is to examine the *approach* taken with regard to a particular sub-criterion. Is it sound, with a clear rationale and well-defined and developed processes, and does it focus on stakeholder needs? Also, is it integrated, supporting policy and strategy, and linked to other approaches as appropriate?

The second step is *deployment*, in particular whether the approach has been implemented and if so whether it has been implemented in some areas but not others, and also whether the approach is deployed in a structured way.

Assessment and review is the third and final step in scoring enablers. The organization needs to demonstrate that it is regularly measuring the effectiveness of the approach and the way that deployment is carried out; that learning activities are used to identify and share best practice and opportunities for improvement; and that output from measurement and learning activities is analysed and used to identify, prioritize, plan and implement improvements.

In scoring each element, the assessment team will be looking to see what evidence there is in support of the organization's statements. If such evidence is anecdotal only then a fairly low score will be given. To get a high score there must be clear or comprehensive evidence. In developing a final score for each sub-criterion, simple arithmetic averaging of the scores for approach, deployment and assessment and review is normally used. However, in some cases (e.g. a poor approach widely deployed) subjective judgement is used to give a more reliable score for the sub-criterion. To make sure that the actual numerical score given is comparable with that of other organizations it is important that the assessment team receives appropriate training from qualified EFQM assessors. In developing a final score for each enabler, each of the sub-criteria for an individual enabler are equally weighted within that criterion.

Carrying out a self-assessment

A full self-assessment involves, for each sub-criterion of the model, examining the organization's strengths and areas for improvement (AFIs), as well as completing a scoring sheet for each sub-criterion. There are however a number of ways an organization can carry out a self-assessment based on the Excellence Model, all of which involve some training of staff in the use of the model. The choice will depend on the time and resources available. For example, it is possible to examine each of the nine criteria without examining

Attribute	A	B	C	D	E
Approach (a) Sound: • Approach has a clear rationale • There are well defined and developed processes • Approach focuses on stakeholder needs (b) Integrated: • Approach supports policy and strategy • Approach is linked to other approaches as appropriate	No evidence or anecdotal No evidence or anecdotal	Some evidence Some evidence	Evidence Evidence	Clear evidence Clear evidence	Comprehensive evidence Comprehensive evidence
Deployment (a) Implemented: • Approach is implemented (b) Systematic: • Approach is deployed in a structured way	No evidence or anecdotal No evidence or anecdotal	Implemented in about 1/4 of relevant areas Some evidence	Implemented in about 1/2 of relevant areas Evidence	Implemented in about 3/4 of relevant areas Clear evidence	Implemented in all relevant areas Comprehensive evidence
Assessment and review (a) Measurement: • Regular measurement of the effectiveness of the approach and deployment (b) Learning: • Learning activities are used to identify and share best practice and improvement opportunities (c) Improvement: • Output from measurement and learning is analysed and used to identify, prioritise, plan and implement improvements	No evidence or anecdotal No evidence or anecdotal No evidence or anecdotal	Some evidence Some evidence Some evidence	Evidence Evidence Evidence	Clear evidence Clear evidence Clear evidence	Comprehensive evidence Comprehensive evidence Comprehensive evidence

Figure 4.7 Scoring enablers with the EFQM Excellence Model
Source: Based on EFQM (1999). © EFQM. The EFQM Excellence Model is a registered trademark.

each sub-criteria individually. The model should be used flexibly. The aim is to improve services, not to produce a comprehensive document.

There are a number of approaches to performing an assessment. These include the following, beginning with the least resource intensive.

A *matrix chart approach*, through which team members first give an individual rating based on a matrix consisting of a number of statements of achievements and then meets with a facilitator to develop a consensus. This can be carried out in a two-hour session. Figure 4.8 shows the matrix used by Excellence North West (2000) in their Marques of Excellence programme. In addition to producing some insights for the organization, this approach provides a very good introduction to the model. However, the scores given are typically very optimistic and cannot be compared easily with other units or departments. Nevertheless, for a small investment this exercise is a good starting point. I have personally found it very useful when working with organizations that are newly created out of two different cultures. It is not too intrusive at this delicate stage, but serves as a useful focus for dialogue.

A *workshop approach* where staff meet with trained assessors who act as facilitators for the process. A typical example is to hold a one-day training workshop for senior managers. As well as explaining how the model works, the assessors will give the managers an opportunity to practise self-assessment in a limited way, often by concentrating on one element, such as customer results, and identifying some strengths and AFIs. Individual managers then agree to sponsor a particular criterion and then work with other staff in their area to collect relevant information. The team then come together in another workshop (two days later would be ideal) and the assessor helps them to form a consensus view of the organization's strengths and AFIs. An action plan is then produced to address the AFIs.

A *pro-forma approach* (or workbook method as it is sometimes known). This invites staff to identify strengths, AFIs and evidence provided for each criterion or sub-criterion. Pro-formas contain details of each sub-criteria at the top of the form, while the body of the pro-forma has headings such as strengths, supporting evidence and AFIs. These pro-formas can be completed on a team or individual basis and a consensus obtained in a workshop setting.

A *software-based questionnaire approach*. One such software package is RapidScore, available from the British Quality Foundation. This approach allows easy benchmarking against other organizations.

An *award simulation approach* which involves writing a submission document as if for the British Quality Award.

Self-assessment and business planning

Self-assessment by itself will achieve little. It is the actions that result from the self-assessment which provide the main benefits. Indeed, if the outcomes of the self-assessment are ignored this is more likely to set back the process of quality improvement.

Organisational self analysis chart

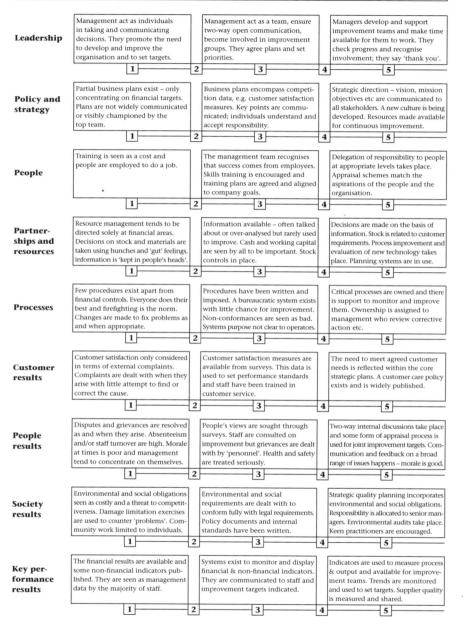

Leadership	Management act as individuals in taking and communicating decisions. They promote the need to develop and improve the organisation and to set targets.	Management act as a team, ensure two-way open communication, become involved in improvement groups. They agree plans and set priorities.	Managers develop and support improvement teams and make time available for them to work. They check progress and recognise involvement; they say 'thank you'.
	1 ─── **2**	─── **3** ─── **4**	─── **5**
Policy and strategy	Partial business plans exist – only concentrating on financial targets. Plans are not widely communicated or visibly championed by the top team.	Business plans encompass competition data, e.g. customer satisfaction measures. Key points are communicated; individuals understand and accept responsibility.	Strategic direction – vision, mission objectives etc are communicated to all stakeholders. A new culture is being developed. Resources made available for continuous improvement.
	1 ─── **2**	─── **3** ─── **4**	─── **5**
People	Training is seen as a cost and people are employed to do a job.	The management team recognises that success comes from employees. Skills training is encouraged and training plans are agreed and aligned to company goals.	Delegation of responsibility to people at appropriate levels takes place. Appraisal schemes match the aspirations of the people and the organisation.
	1 ─── **2**	─── **3** ─── **4**	─── **5**
Partnerships and resources	Resource management tends to be directed solely at financial areas. Decisions on stock and materials are taken using hunches and 'gut' feelings, information is 'kept in people's heads'.	Information available – often talked about or over-analysed but rarely used to improve. Cash and working capital are seen by all to be important. Stock controls in place.	Decisions are made on the basis of information. Stock is related to customer requirements. Process improvement and evaluation of new technology takes place. Planning systems are in use.
	1 ─── **2**	─── **3** ─── **4**	─── **5**
Processes	Few procedures exist apart from financial controls. Everyone does their best and firefighting is the norm. Changes are made to fix problems as and when appropriate.	Procedures have been written and imposed. A bureaucratic system exists with little chance for improvement. Non-conformances are seen as bad. Systems purpose not clear to operators.	Critical processes are owned and there is support to monitor and improve them. Ownership is assigned to management who review corrective action etc.
	1 ─── **2**	─── **3** ─── **4**	─── **5**
Customer results	Customer satisfaction only considered in terms of external complaints. Complaints are dealt with when they arise with little attempt to find or correct the cause.	Customer satisfaction measures are available from surveys. This data is used to set performance standards and staff have been trained in customer service.	The need to meet agreed customer needs is reflected within the core strategic plans. A customer care policy exists and is widely published.
	1 ─── **2**	─── **3** ─── **4**	─── **5**
People results	Disputes and grievances are resolved as and when they arise. Absenteeism and/or staff turnover are high. Morale at times is poor and management tend to concentrate on themselves.	People's views are sought through surveys. Staff are consulted on improvement but grievances are dealt with by 'personnel'. Health and safety are treated seriously.	Two-way internal discussions take place and some form of appraisal process is used for joint improvement targets. Communication and feedback on a broad range of issues happens – morale is good.
	1 ─── **2**	─── **3** ─── **4**	─── **5**
Society results	Environmental and social obligations seen as costly and a threat to competitiveness. Damage limitation exercises are used to counter 'problems'. Community work limited to individuals.	Environmental and social requirements are dealt with to conform fully with legal requirements. Policy documents and internal standards have been written.	Strategic quality planning incorporates environmental and social obligations. Responsibility is allocated to senior managers. Environmental audits take place. Keen practitioners are encouraged.
	1 ─── **2**	─── **3** ─── **4**	─── **5**
Key performance results	The financial results are available and some non-financial indicators published. They are seen as management data by the majority of staff.	Systems exist to monitor and display financial & non-financial indicators. They are communicated to staff and improvement targets indicated.	Indicators are used to measure process & output and available for improvement teams. Trends are monitored and used to set targets. Supplier quality is measured and shared.
	1 ─── **2**	─── **3** ─── **4**	─── **5**

Figure 4.8 Matrix chart from Excellence North West
Source: Excellence North West (2000).

Starting with Leadership, read all the statements across the page and choose and circle the number you feel best reflects the situation within your organisation. Multiply the number you have chosen by the factor shown and enter your score in the box on the right. Repeat the exercise for the other eight criteria and total your scores to produce a grand total.

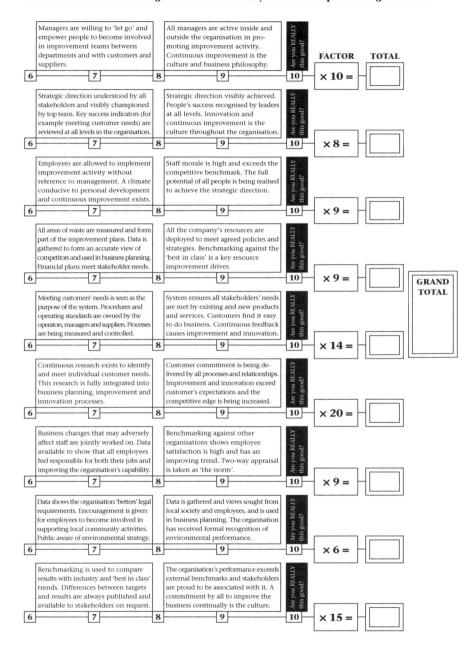

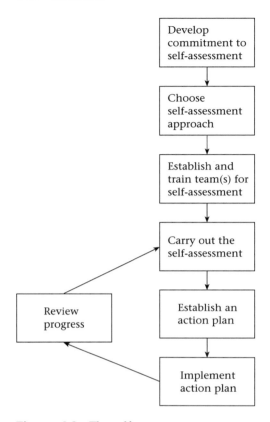

Figure 4.9 The self-assessment process

Self-assessment is only one stage in the process (see Figure 4.9). Following the self-assessment, it is important to establish an action plan covering the areas that need addressing together with priorities. The next stage is to implement the plan ensuring that sufficient resources are provided and that implementation is monitored. Progress can then be reviewed and a further self-assessment conducted.

NCH, a large UK voluntary child care organization, looked at this the other way round. They wanted to introduce the Excellence Model, but were concerned about the heavy workloads already borne by staff. Camilla Wood, Senior Quality Assurance Officer at NCH, says, 'it proved helpful to relate the outcome of the self-assessment to business planning, in that the process could help to identify areas for development which the plan needed to address. Since the business plan had to be done, the self-assessment became an aid to its achievement, rather than an additional burden' (Quality Standards Task Group 2001).

Implementing the Excellence Model in social care

The following list of suggestions was developed by the British Quality Foundation's Social Care Group in a seminar in June 1999.

- Involve the front line in self-assessment and improvement (everyone, not just the 'assessment team').
- Engage people through personal motivation.
- Make it real: use language people can relate to.
- Relate the model to external pressures and business drivers.
- Focus on the user perspective.
- Stop talking about the model and start talking about the results that are important to the staff group and to the organization.
- Start with the model as a framework for thinking and reflecting.
- People results and management of people are often good starting points in talking about the model. However, it is important to ensure that all the parts are dealt with.
- Get early wins so that staff can see the difference and that the effort is worth it.
- Get staff and managers to think 'What's in it for me?': the satisfaction of demonstrating success, better job security, team membership, pride in themselves and the organization, increased involvement and influence, personal recognition and kudos.
- Get leadership to consider how the use of the model can be sustained. Get leaders actively involved.
- Get the use of the model into individual staff member's development portfolio so credit is given.
- Build the use of the model into the regular processes of the organization. Tie into what is already going on and into business planning.
- Stop and deal with the notion that the model is an extra burden which is just another thing hard-pressed staff have to do.
- Get some excitement into the notion of measurement. We want to know where we are so we can put energy into the right area. Remember that some social care staff have a negative reaction to numbers.
- Make the quality journey and use of the model fun and enjoyable.

Case studies

Three case studies are included in this section: one in health, one in a local authority social services department and one from the voluntary sector.

South Tees Acute Hospitals NHS Trust colposcopy clinic

South Tees Acute Hospitals NHS Trust (STAHT) was one of the pioneers of the use of the Excellence Model in health care. It began using the model in

Table 4.3 Improvements in results at South Tees Colposcopy Clinic

	Before	*After*
Time to generate appointment	13.5 days	24 hours (for GP) 48 hours (for patient)
Wait for first appointment	13 weeks	2–4 weeks
Consultation time	10 minutes	30 minutes
Did not attend rate	20%	10%

1995, piloting it in selected areas within the hospital, and since then the model has been used in a wide variety of areas within the Trust. Two major success factors in their successful implementation of the model were the commitment from the start of the Trust's chief executive, Bill Murray, and the involvement of key clinicians as well as senior managers in the use of the model.

This is the context in which the model was introduced in the colposcopy clinic within the Trust's Division of Women and Children. Colposcopy is essentially the follow-up service for women whose cervical smears gave a positive test result. The clinic had 750 new referrals per year and was very effective from a clinical point of view. However, staff and patients were frustrated with the way it worked. All the staff involved in the process, led by the consultant Stuart Hutchinson, met together with a local GP to review and redesign the process. They began by measuring customer results. These included 13.5 days to generate an appointment, a 13-week wait for a first appointment and an 8-week wait for a second appointment. The process was redesigned based on what patients wanted from the service, while also taking note of the impact on staff. Discussions with GPs also took place to ensure improved processes for referral and recall for consultation.

The impact of the changes made, which included direct referral from cytology and a 'see and treat' service for certain patients, is shown in Table 4.3. The time to generate an appointment was initially reduced to 24 hours, however it was found that since many GPs only open their mail after morning surgery, some patients went to see their GP having seen the results to find the GP was unaware of them. Instead therefore the clinic changed the time to 24 hours for the GP and 48 hours for patients. The wait for the first appointment also reduced dramatically. Under the new system the 'did not attend' rate has halved and the number of unnecessary repeat smears was reduced by 100 per cent. From the patients' point of view, not only has the process been speeded up, reducing needless anxiety, but also the consultation time has increased giving them a better service all round. Moreover, staff satisfaction and the satisfaction of referring GPs with the new service are both very high. Further detail on the use of the Excellence Model in South Tees is given in Stahr *et al.* (2000).

Cheshire social services

Cheshire social services began implementing the Excellence Model in 1995 and in the first year piloted about six self-assessments based on the model. A variety of teams ranging from the management and delivery of services to older people, to teams looking at training and support were involved, each team being asked to assess its performance against the nine criteria of the model.

The method of self-assessment varied from a one and a half day workshop based on people's perception of the organization, to a more comprehensive assessment based on information obtained via interviews, questionnaires and analysis carried out over a period of three months. In all cases, the self-assessments were followed by each team prioritizing the areas for improvement and implementing detailed action plans to improve the service. These pilots were very successful and were followed by further initiatives based on the model.

In 1996, several short-life groups were set up across the organization looking at different aspects of social services (e.g. the delivery of adult, older people and children services). The nine criteria were used to trigger key questions about the future. For example, what was the vision for the organization in the future? Were their policies and strategies the right ones? What would the culture of the organization look like in the future? What skills would managers and staff need? What results did they want to achieve in relation to financial and non-financial targets, customer and employee satisfaction and the views of the people of Cheshire?

Cheshire social services used the model to identify the critical processes. These included operational processes (assessing needs and purchasing care, delivering care and managing risk) and support processes. The latter included priority setting, financial and people management, specifying and managing contracts, and managing communications with customers, staff and other organizations. These processes were analysed to make sure that they were well-managed, efficient, effective, customer-orientated and added value.

Painter and Johnson (1997) conclude: 'The use of the Excellence Model has helped Cheshire Social Services to review its internal workings, overcome barriers to effective performance, and look towards the future. It has been a key driver in relation to organisational change and development, and a useful management tool in the process of building and maintaining a learning organisation'.

Thames Reach

Thames Reach provides a range of street outreach, resettlement, community support and accommodation services to rough sleepers in London. It has around 96 full-time staff, 15 part-time staff and 20 volunteers. Rebecca Pritchard, Housing Services Manager, who helped lead the work using the Excellence Model, says that they chose the model because of its emphasis on self-assessment and continuous improvement, and that it seemed flexible enough to use across the whole organization. Also, they felt they could derive tangible benefits even with limited resources.

They began by giving a presentation to Thames Reach's board and were successful in gaining support for using the model. They then established a group of staff, including both main grade workers and managers, who would represent each service within the organization. The first session was an introduction to the model and team members decided to focus on the customer results criterion, discussing who the stakeholders were and what information they had which would provide evidence of customer results.

Team members were then given a simple self-assessment questionnaire, based on one developed by the National Council for Voluntary Organizations. As well as completing the questionnaires, they were asked to meet with staff in their service area to identify some strengths and AFIs for customer results.

At the next meeting, one service area volunteered to be a guinea-pig for the scoring process. It was stressed that while scoring helped focus on the type of evidence presented, it was less important than identifying AFIs. Following this session, teams were asked to produce similar results.

Among the AFIs identified from the analysis of the customer results criterion were:

- develop link workers between day centres and outreach services to improve clients' understanding of, and access to, the service;
- develop client care plan reviews so they offer an explicit opportunity for clients' views and perceptions of the service to be recorded;
- develop organization-wide mechanisms for responding to complaints and feedback from clients, and ensure there is regular feedback and analysis of all such information;
- develop statistics and measures that will help describe the service and the process of resettlement for new clients;
- develop mechanisms for receiving feedback from referral agencies.

Thames Reach felt that due to time constraints, they could focus only on one model criterion at a time. They recognized however that by adopting this approach there was a risk that they could lose sight of the links between enablers and results. They did feel, however, that using the Excellence Model was worthwhile and that many of the AFIs would not otherwise have been identified. They decided to continue with the use of the model and also to take action on the AFIs identified.

Rebecca Pritchard recommends the following, based on their experiences in using the model (Quality Standards Task Group 2001):

- Keep it simple and build up gradually.
- Be realistic about the amount of resources (especially time) you can afford to dedicate to the process. If you overstretch, it will be harder to keep up any momentum.
- Make the commitment and be aware that you will need to have senior management support to ensure the work is a priority.

- A lot of the success of the model is in changing the way people think, looking for links between results and enablers outside formal self-assessment, and realizing that the model *can* make a difference.
- Don't get hung up about scoring in the early stages. Ours were not good, but we felt that using the model would genuinely help improve our services, even if some areas of the scoring regime were still not fully addressed.
- Avoid developing systems for their own sake – select the AFIs that are meaningful and add value to your services, not your scores alone.
- Put most of your energy into delivering improvements, and try to avoid creating more paperwork – that way you can sell the model to (hard-pressed) staff, and ensure real commitment and benefits accrue to all your stakeholders.

Using the model if limited time is available

Many organizations in health and social care would like to gain the benefits of the Excellence Model but do not feel they have time to do a full self-assessment. To conclude the chapter, here is my recommended approach in such situations:

1 Run a short workshop with staff using a matrix approach, getting a feel for the organization's main strengths and areas for improvement (AFIs).
2 Focus on *customer results*. Find out what users and other key stakeholders want from the service and identify how well it meets their needs. Also look at *key performance results*.
3 Next, draw a detailed process flow diagram (Chapter 8) showing how *processes* are carried out at present. Then, working with the team, identify whether each step adds value to the user and see how the process can be improved. Be prepared to radically alter the process if necessary.
4 While looking at the process, identify how well the organization is doing on the other enablers. This may indicate that *policy and strategy* are unclear, or that *leadership* and/or *partnerships and resources* need attention. In all cases identify AFIs.
5 Next, look at *people results*. What do these indicate about how well *people* are developed, motivated and recognized? Do they provide guidance on other enablers that need to be addressed? Again identify AFIs. Also look at *society results*.
6 Look at the performance measures available. Can they be improved? In particular, do they measure the right things? Are all aspects of importance to users included?
7 Develop an action plan addressing the areas for improvement identified and carry it out.
8 By now, managers, staff and hopefully users will have seen many benefits from using the model. While the momentum is there, discuss the next steps in using the model.

CHAPTER five

Leadership, policy and strategy

The critical importance in the Excellence Model of both leadership, and policy and strategy, can be seen from Figure 5.1 which shows how the different elements relate to one another for planning purposes (as opposed to self-assessment). Leadership drives policy and strategy and together they set a clear strategic direction for the organization. These, along with people management, and partnerships and resources, interact with processes to improve results for all the organization's stakeholders – patients, service users, carers, partner organizations, staff, society and government.

Many senior managers in all sectors of the economy have 'seen the light' about quality. They are convinced of its benefits to their organization. They understand what TQM is and what is required to achieve it. However, rather than tackle the issues head-on, they find it much easier to show *some* commitment to quality, to make *some* quality improvements, perhaps in the areas that most need addressing, and to make *some* move towards involving their staff in the quality improvement process. They are, however, understandably nervous about making the changes required to transform the culture so that organizational excellence becomes the standard.

Most managers in Europe and North America, whether in health and social care or elsewhere, try to manage by *management by control*. Each manager, beginning at the top, is given certain goals for the next year – for example to reduce costs or increase profit by 10 per cent. This goal then gets passed to all division heads who in turn pass it down the line to each departmental head. In a manufacturing company, for example, the marketing department may be told to increase sales by 10 per cent, operations to reduce costs by 5 per cent, engineering to get products into production 10 per cent faster, while purchasing is told to reduce its costs by 5 per cent etc. Eventually, at lower levels, these goals become quotas or work

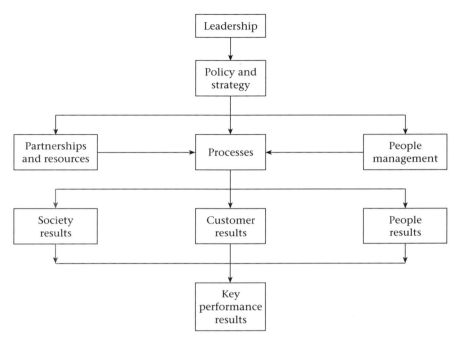

Figure 5.1 Relationship between different elements of the EFQM Excellence Model for business planning

standards. Furthermore, financial and other rewards are typically given for meeting these internally generated controls rather than for providing a product or service that meets the needs of the organization's customers or users. Where individual goals are set without a long-term larger purpose there will always be conflict. Each department is interested in meeting its quota. The purchasing department, for example, can meet its quota by ordering cheaper, poorer quality products, but this will not be in the company's best interests.

If a social work team is told to increase its number of assessments by 20 per cent with the same processes and fewer resources, either the quality of the assessments will reduce or the social workers will become even more stressed (or both). However, if the manager involved social workers and users in looking at the existing processes used, identifying areas where things could be speeded up and costs reduced without detriment to service users, there would be real opportunities to improve quality all round. As Feigenbaum (1991) says, 'Getting quality results is not a short-term instant-pudding way to improve competitiveness; implementing total quality management requires hands-on, continuous leadership'.

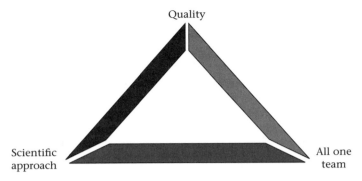

Figure 5.2 The Joiner triangle

Total quality leadership (TQL)

The alternative to management control, according to Brian Joiner and Peter Scholtes (1988), is total quality leadership (TQL). This aims to create an environment that allows and encourages everyone to contribute to the organization by developing the skills needed to scientifically study and constantly improve every process by which work is accomplished. The essence of TQL is illustrated in what is known as the 'Joiner triangle' – see Figure 5.2.

The focus is on *quality* – the quality of every product and service and the quality of every process. To achieve this higher quality, every process, beginning with the most important, is studied using a *scientific approach*. Processes are described with flow charts, problems are identified, the root causes of problems are determined through careful research and new systems are developed. The other requirement for TQL is to create an environment of *all one team*. Everyone throughout the organization must learn to work together to improve processes and to execute them with efficiency. However, for all employees to be committed to the organization and its customers, the organization must be committed to them.

There are a number of principles of quality leadership for health and social care (based on Scholtes 1998):

- focus on patients, carers and service users;
- obsession with quality;
- supporting and empowering employees;
- using statistical and other methods to understand the process;
- unity of purpose;
- encouraging employees to look for improvements in the system;
- teamwork;
- continued education and training.

Characteristics of effective leaders

The field of human resource management is very rich in this area. Robbins and Finley (1996) identify the following characteristics of effective leaders:

- They project energy, demonstrating enthusiasm and commitment.
- They are involved, involving and empowering of others.
- They assist evolution and change by ensuring that everyone is motivated and understands what's in it for them.
- They persuade and persevere in their attempts to get resources for their teams, removing obstacles and clearing a path.
- They look beyond the obvious researching and evaluating information. They take time to collect all the facts.
- They maintain perspective and don't lose sight of the goal-keeping visions: stretching enough to motivate people but not too stretching that people lose interest.
- They encourage everyone in the team to learn, avoiding pockets of knowledge so that if one member were to leave then the team would not suffer.
- They are good at targeting their own and others' energies on opportunities for success.
- They foster task linkage with others. They help to break down the barriers with other parts of the organization. They influence cooperative action with other groups.

It is also useful to compare Robbins and Finley's list with some research commissioned by the Industrial Society to find out what organizations wanted their leaders to be like in the future and what people rated as important in defining good leadership behaviour. The main findings were as follows (Couldstone 1999):

- Organizations don't want bosses; they want leaders who will make the right space for people to perform well without having to be watched over.
- Organizations want flat structures where people can be trusted to work with minimal supervision.
- Organizations want a wide range of people to be able to take a lead and lead a project, step into a leadership role when necessary and consistently behave in a responsible way.
- Organizations want a culture where people can be responsive to customer demands and agile in the face of changing technology.

These findings are as relevant to health and social care as to other organizations, as the following quote from David Fillingham makes clear:

Transforming the NHS requires leaders who can:

- develop a vision of the future for patient care and plans for achieving that future;

Table 5.1 Managers and leaders

Managers	Leaders
Make plans for the future (on paper)	Have a vision for the future
Manage by objectives	Use participative management
Give lip-service to quality	Produce exemplary quality
Sell to customers	Provide service to customers
Cut costs	Create less waste through better processes
Control people and things through systems	Develop people's talents, control things through systems
Reward conformance, punish deviation	Reward effort, skill development and innovation
Maintain status quo	Look to continuous improvement

Source: Bennis and Nanus (1985).

- create teams and coalitions and gain the intense co-operation needed to implement radical change;
- motivate staff and inspire action to overcome major barriers to change.

(Modernisation Agency 2001)

One distinction which is particularly useful here is that between management and leadership. Management is predominantly activity-based and is concerned with matters such as planning, budgeting, organizing and problem solving. Leadership on the other hand involves dealing with people rather than things – creating a sense of direction, communicating the vision and energizing, inspiring and motivating. The main differences between managers and leaders are given in Table 5.1, which is based on Bennis and Nanus (1985). Moving away from the characteristics in the left-hand column towards those in the right is a prerequisite for TQM. Rajan and Van Eupen (1996) summarize the differences as follows: 'Management is about now, leadership is about the future; one implements goals, the other sets them; one relies on control, the other inspires trust; one deals in rational processes, the other in emotional horizons'.

Cook (1992) gives the following list of characteristics of a good 'service-style leader'. They should:

- be a good listener;
- encourage teamwork and good communication;
- delegate responsibility;
- require and recognize excellence;
- encourage problem solving;
- request and welcome feedback;
- constantly seek out ideas and improvements;

- engender trust;
- be open and honest in their dealings.

Leadership styles

Vroom and Yago (1988) identify three different management styles: auto-cratic, consultative and group. These are described in Table 5.2. The import-ance of this classification is not to imply that one style is best for all decisions, but to highlight the differences and make leaders consider which style is most appropriate for a particular problem. For example, a senior clinical consultant may find that a more autocratic style is best when operating on an emergency patient, while in a weekly review meeting or a clinical governance review the consultative or group styles work best. John Clark, who headed the company BET until its takeover by Rentokil, believes that leaders also need to adapt their leadership style to the phases of the organizational life cycle: 'When you're fighting for the survival of the business, action-orientation, enthusiasm, leading from the front – all these are critical factors . . . Then in the new phase you must be more thoughtful, more strategic. Above all what matters is continually being able to look afresh at a business situation' (quoted in Trapp 1997).

Table 5.2 Leadership styles

Style	Characteristics
Autocratic	Leader makes the decisions for the group, either using just information available to the leader at that time or possibly also using information generated from subordinates.
Consultative	Leader determines problem definition and shares the ideas with subordinates either individually or in a group. Leader makes decision which may or may not reflect subordinate input.
Group	Leader determines problem definition and shares the ideas with subordinates in a group. The group develops alternative solutions to the problem and attempts are made to elicit a consensus of agreement. The leader role here is one of facilitation and the group makes the decision to which both the leader and the group are committed.

Source: Vroom and Yago (1988).

Vroom and Yago (1988) suggest that when reflecting on their leadership style, managers should ask themselves the following questions:

- How important is the technical quality of this decision?
- How important is subordinate commitment to this decision?
- Do you have sufficient information to make a high-quality decision?

- Is the problem well structured?
- If you make the decision yourself, how likely is it that your subordinates would be committed?
- Do subordinates share the organizational goals to be attained in solving this problem?
- Is conflict among subordinates likely over preferred solutions?
- Do subordinates have sufficient information to make a high-quality decision?
- Are the costs involved in bringing together geographically dispersed subordinates prohibitive?
- How important is it to make the decision quickly?
- How important is it to you to increase the opportunities for subordinate development?

Leadership competencies

Scholtes (1999) identifies six competencies which are required for effective leadership:

- The ability to think in terms of systems and knowing how to lead systems. For an organizational system to function properly, it must have a clear, constant, well-integrated purpose – which in turn requires effective leadership.
- The ability to understand the variability of work in planning and problem solving. Less than 3 per cent of leaders understand this. Many see trends where there are no trends and miss trends that exist.
- Understanding how we learn, develop and improve, and leading true learning and improvement. Scholtes cautions against simplistic solutions to complex problems, quoting Albert Einstein: 'We must make things as simple as possible, and not any simpler'.
- Understanding people and why they behave as they do. Many leaders do not understand about motivation, which is not about 'a stick and a carrot. It is not something infused, like a bone marrow. Rather, it is a relationship nurtured over time'.
- Understanding the interdependence and interaction between systems, variation, learning and human behaviour: knowing how each affects the others.
- Giving vision, meaning, direction and focus to the organization. This involves continually reminding people of the organization's purpose, aims and priorities. It is also vital to lead by example.

British Telecom identify a number of aspects of good leadership: a manager's personal style, direction setting, the ability to get results, managing relationships and leadership of change. They also identify seven core management competencies for effective leadership – see Figure 5.3.

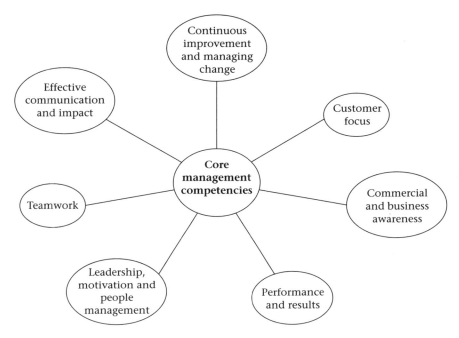

Figure 5.3 Core management competencies for BT

Leadership of change

> There is nothing more difficult or perilous than to take the lead in the introduction of change.
>
> (Machiavelli)

There are two aspects to delivering excellence in health and social care. One is identifying with staff, users and partners where the organization or service needs to go in order to deliver excellence, and the other is making sure that the changes required actually take place. The second aspect is by far the most difficult. It has been said that seven out of ten projects fail, not because of a lack of good ideas, but because of a failure to implement and sustain them. The way quality management and organizational excellence is introduced and implemented in an organization is a vital factor in its eventual success. Managers need to be very aware of potential difficulties in implementation and how best to overcome them, and in particular understand the issues surrounding the management of change.

Figure 5.4, based on Munchi (1992), illustrates common problems in implementing and sustaining an ongoing quality management programme. These are categorized according to whether they are due to management systems, senior management, employee attitudes or work methods.

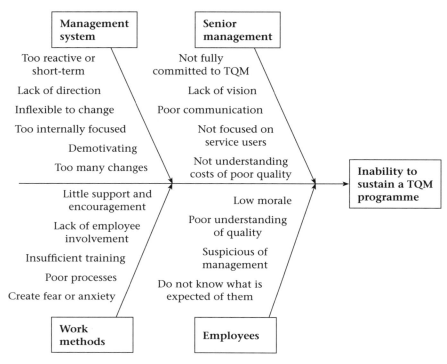

Figure 5.4   Barriers to the successful implementation of TQM programmes
Source: Haigh and Morris (2001).

Another difficulty is that while the benefits of change for the organization may be clear, not everyone will see it as being in their personal self-interest! As Thomas (1994) puts it: 'There are those who buy into the quality message with an intensity that borders on the obsessive and those who eschew it with equal vigour. In the middle are the non-committed, waiting to see what will happen in the long run'.

In order to increase the proportion of people who are positive about change, it is useful to identify the extent to which the organization, perhaps subconsciously, inhibits the desired response from its staff and stifles innovation. In such an environment people are likely to distrust the management and not respond positively to change. If, for example, the existing culture tends to regard any idea from below with suspicion, expresses criticism freely but withholds praise, treats identification of problems as signs of failure and springs changes on people unexpectedly, these issues need to be tackled head-on: 'Change is always a threat when it's done to me or imposed on me, whether I like it or not. But it's an opportunity if it's done by me. It's my chance to contribute and be recognised. That is the simple key to all of this: make it an opportunity for people and reward them for it' (Kanter 1983).

There are a number of important principles in implementing change. These include:

- Involving people at all levels in the change process as early as possible.
- Working together as a team.
- Communicating as never before.
- Openness and transparency.
- Acknowledgement of external drivers – for example, where the main reason for change is a directive from top management or central government.
- Generosity in success, giving credit where credit is due.
- Inclusive approaches.
- Being flexible – knowing where the organization is heading but allowing for detours where they are needed. Flexibility is also needed regarding the *pace* of change.

In terms of the last point, about the pace of change, Oakland (1995) identifies two basic approaches to implementation of quality programmes:

- the 'blitz' approach in which the whole organization is suddenly exposed very rapidly to TQM, with mass education and plenty of hype;
- the slow, planned, purposeful approach causing a gradual change to take place.

The blitz approach has been tried in a number of organizations. However, this typically gives rise to a number of problems, partly because employees do not have time to establish whether top management is really committed or whether the initiative will be short-lived. There will be a feeling that change is being forced through without the degree of consensus that quality management requires. In Oakland's (1995) words, 'some organisations have suffered indigestion by trying to swallow the "elephant" whole, instead of a bite each time'.

The slow, purposeful approach might seem to take too long, but delivering excellence is a journey and must be seen as a long-term investment in the organization.

Glanfield (2001), drawing on research by Pettigrew (1998) summarizes some lessons from research on the leadership of change:

- see change as a long journey, not a short-term episode;
- promote coherence across the (inevitably) multi-faceted change agenda;
- emphasize what will *not* change and create zones of continuity and comfort;
- promote customization – local solutions for local people;
- find opportunities for leaders to marry top-down pressures with bottom-up concerns;
- see change as a political process; operate inclusive and voluntary principles and create conditions for self-organization.

Developing a learning culture

A key challenge of leadership of change is to develop a learning culture in the organization. There are two main aspects to developing a learning culture: being able to learn from mistakes (avoiding a blame culture) and learning from others. These relate closely to two of the core values of the Excellence Model: management by fact and continuous learning. The concept of a learning organization is very relevant here. Senge (1990) defines learning organizations as 'organisations where people continually expand their capacity to create the results they truly desire, where new and expansive patterns of thinking are nurtured, where collective aspiration is set free, and where people are continually learning to learn together'. To become a learning organization there needs to be 'systematic problem solving, experimentation with new approaches, learning from best practice elsewhere, and transferring knowledge quickly and efficiently throughout the organisation' (Garvin 1993).

Iles and Sutherland (2001) give five main characteristics of the learning organization:

- *Structure*: flat managerial hierarchies that enhance opportunities for employee involvement, supporting teamwork, strong lateral relations and networking across organizational and departmental boundaries.
- *Information systems*: facilitating rapid acquisition, processing and sharing of rich, complex information to support effective knowledge management.
- *Human resource practices*: focusing on provision and support of individual learning, with appropriate appraisal and reward systems.
- *Organizational culture*: promoting openness and creativity; encouraging people to try new things and to learn from mistakes.
- *Leadership*: leaders need to demonstrate the openness, risk-taking and reflection necessary for learning, and to communicate this vision to others.

An Organisation with a Memory (Department of Health 2000a), which is concerned with learning from adverse events in the NHS, identifies three key areas in which the NHS falls short of being a learning organization:

- *There is too often a 'blame' culture.* When things go wrong, the knee-jerk reaction is to find someone to blame and discipline them, rather than looking at the root cause of the problem, which may be due to poor management practice, poor communication or poor systems. Ann Tucker, a carer, is quoted in the *Observer* newspaper (Tucker 2001) as follows: 'There's a culture of blame in both medicine and the social services, and where there's blame there's the need to be defensive – and that's all a distraction from the real work of looking after the ill person'.
- *No account is taken of near misses.* Research in aviation and elsewhere indicates that for every major incident there may be several hundred near misses. The NHS is poor in learning from adverse events that do not result

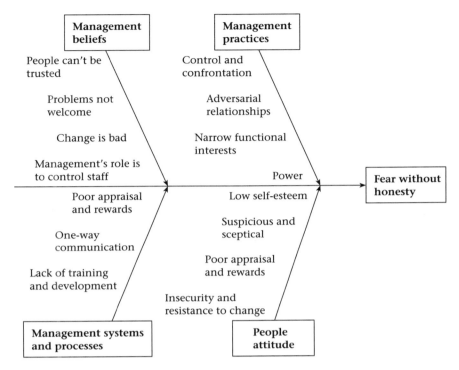

Figure 5.5 Deficiencies in management
Source: Lowe and McBean (1989).

in significant harm, but these provide a rich source of information for preventing serious problems.

- *There is little culture of individual self-appraisal.* Unless NHS professionals acknowledge that perfection is not always attained, both to themselves and their colleagues, there is little opportunity for learning from mistakes or continuous improvement.

These issues are by no means confined to the NHS. In a survey of quality managers who had ongoing TQM programmes begun in 1989, Haigh and Morris (2001) found that 73 per cent agreed that their organizations had a tendency to deal with specific episodes of bad quality rather than remove the underlying causes. Figure 5.5, based on Lowe and McBean (1989), is a cause and effect diagram illustrating the deficiencies in management in both the manufacturing and service sectors of western economies which lead to a climate of 'fear without honesty'. This can be caused by management beliefs (e.g. a belief that staff cannot be trusted), by poor management practices (e.g. management by control), by poor systems and processes or by poor people attitudes.

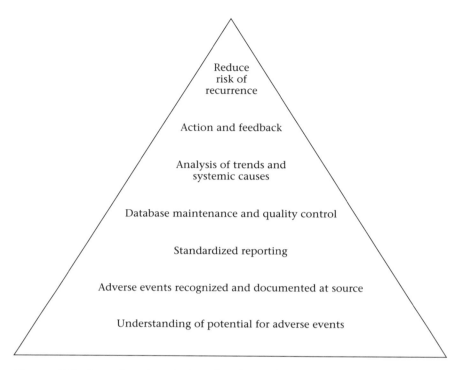

Figure 5.6 Some key steps in learning from adverse events
Source: Department of Health (2000a).

To address these deficiencies, the expert group set up by the Department of Health (2000a) identified seven steps for learning from adverse events – see Figure 5.6.

In addition to learning from mistakes, a learning organization develops ways of sharing best practice and learning from other organizations. As the NHS Plan says: 'Spreading best practice in the NHS however is often slow and ad hoc' (National Health Service 2000). The *Quality Strategy for Social Care* (Department of Health 2000b) goes further: 'One of the main reasons for inconsistencies in the quality of service across the country is the lack of reliable evidence about what works best in social care. There is simply not enough rigorous information on ways of raising the quality of service, and what information exists is poorly disseminated'.

Developing learning networks is the answer to this and there has been much activity in this area in health and social care in recent years. Learning networks can take a variety of forms. They can be face-to-face meetings, workshops, site visits, e-mail networks or in the form of newsletters or websites. Learning networks need to address a number of key areas including their purpose, who should be invited to participate, whether there will be a coordinator or facilitator, how people will find out about the network and what resources are available to support it. Resources is a key aspect. While it is not always easy taking staff out of day-to-day activities, learning from others is a lot cheaper than reinventing what has been implemented elsewhere. Investing in a learning culture has a clear payback.

The following quote from Lew Platt, chief executive of Hewlett Packard (HP), is very thought-provoking: 'If HP knew what HP knows, we would be three times as profitable'. By the same reasoning, if all health and social care services adopted best practice nationally (or internationally) in their particular service, improvements would be dramatic. Even those units who are seen as adopting best practice on certain aspects will learn from others on other relevant aspects. The potential for improvement as a result of simply sharing knowledge and experience is vast.

This potential for improvement was recognized by NHS Executive Trent (2001) in setting up the Trent Improvement Network 'to enable people in the NHS and its partner organisations to improve services by using what works in their different local contexts'. The Network aims to spread good practices primarily by linking and joining up existing knowledge, experience and practice. It is based on the following four premises:

- sustainable change and improvement is generated by the people who do the job and cannot therefore be imposed;
- most of the know-how and wisdom needed to improve services already exists in the system;
- there is a need to connect up what we know and make it available to all;
- an open organization culture stimulates and encourages improvement.

Visions, missions and core values

A key role of leaders is to develop and facilitate the achievement of the organization's mission and vision, and to identify, with the relevant staff involved, the core values of the service.

The starting point is the vision – where does the organization want to be? This determines the core values and beliefs it wishes to pursue, and together the vision and core values contribute to determining the organization's mission – what it wishes to achieve. This relationship is shown in Figure 5.7.

A vision can be seen as 'an organisation's desirable future state' (Martensen and Dahlgaard 1999) or 'a dream that can be achieved by utilizing the proper means' (Pioneer Electronic Corporation's vision statement). Many people are confused about the difference between a vision and a mission and indeed some organizations use the terms in different ways. The vision is about what an organization would like to be, whereas the mission statement is more practical and concerns what it wishes to achieve. These differences can be seen by examining the vision and mission statements of the Royal

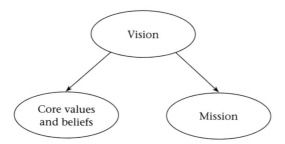

Figure 5.7 The relationship between vision, values and the mission statement

National Institute for the Blind (RNIB). Their vision is: 'A world where people who are blind or partially sighted enjoy the same rights, responsibilities, opportunities and quality of life as people who are sighted'. This statement is very useful in helping staff, blind and partially sighted people, and partner organizations, to identify what the RNIB is about; what they are striving for. It can also be inspiring. However, it is of less use in practical terms as it does not say how the vision might be achieved. This is where the mission statement comes in. The RNIB have a short and long version of their mission (see below). Both of these are clearly consistent with the vision, but provide much more guidance about how that vision can be achieved:

> To challenge blindness by empowering people who are blind or partially sighted, removing the barriers they face and helping to prevent blindness.

> Our Mission is to understand and give a voice to the aspirations and needs of all people who are blind or partially sighted across the UK. We will challenge the disabling effects of blindness by providing services and by ensuring that people who are blind or partially sighted are empowered to get on with their lives. We will challenge society's actions, attitudes and assumptions. Many barriers are put in the path of people who are blind or partially sighted; we will help dismantle them. We will work to ensure that all people avoid preventable sight loss. We will work cooperatively with other organisations in all countries of the UK and worldwide to achieve our Vision.

As mentioned previously, it is useful for an organization to communicate its core values – the principles that should underpin its actions and decisions. The RNIB has six core values: putting the needs of people who are blind and partially sighted first; valuing people (i.e. its staff and volunteers); openness; empowerment; equality; and working together. These core values were used, along with the vision, in determining its mission statements.

Values, vision and mission statements are not just for large organizations. They can also be very useful for an individual department or a small voluntary body. For example, a social care department concerned with children

Table 5.3 Post Office Counters core values and leadership commitment

Core value	Leaders do these things and support others in doing them
Customer focus	Focusing on, understanding and satisfying customer needs
Integrity	Communicating and dealing with others with complete trust, honesty and fairness
Teamwork	Maximizing the contribution individuals can make to the team through effective communication and cooperation and by listening to and supporting each other
Respect	Setting a strong personal example of respect, recognition and active cooperation with others
Innovation	Showing enterprise and welcoming change by taking sensible risks and learning from mistakes
Enthusiasm	Demonstrating a positive spirit and enthusiasm for the mission and driving towards achieving business goals
Professionalism	Working efficiently to get it right first time, managing by fact and eliminating personal prejudice
Continuous improvement	Concentrating on finding solutions rather than simply stating problems, and identifying and acting on improvement opportunities

and families might have an overall aim or mission 'to ensure that children are protected from significant harm and gain maximum life chance benefits by a coordinated range of services being provided for them in the community'. Another example is Sheffield City Council's Family Placement Services Permanence Team which has the following vision: 'to provide safe, stable, secure, loving and capable families for children to grow up in, when they cannot live with their birth families'.

Having developed a mission statement and a set of values, it is important that leaders set an example by following these values and encouraging others to do the same. Table 5.3 shows how Post Office Counters have linked leadership requirements to the organization's core values. Post Office Counters also measure feedback on leaders from team members via a confidential questionnaire with respect to their performance on each of these values.

Implementing policy and strategy

Many organizations have nice-sounding vision and mission statements, which look good in the relevant documents, but the actual policies on the ground may be very different. Implementing policy and strategy is the key to translating the mission and vision into a clear stakeholder-focused strategy, supported by relevant policies, plans, objectives, targets and processes. The following quote from Imai (1986) illustrates the importance of going beyond vision and mission statements and making sure that they are not mere slogans and exhortations:

> To illustrate the need for policy deployment, let us consider the following case: The president of an airline company proclaims that he believes in safety and that his corporate goal is to make sure that safety is maintained throughout the company. This proclamation is prominently featured in the company's quarterly report and its advertising. Let us further suppose that the department managers also swear a firm belief in safety. The catering manager says he believes in safety. The pilots say they believe in safety. The flight crews say they believe in safety. Everyone in the company practices safety. True? Or might everyone simply be paying lip service to the idea of safety?
>
> On the other hand if the president states that safety is company policy and works with his division managers to develop a plan for safety which defines their responsibilities, everyone will have a very specific subject to discuss. Safety will become a real concern. For the manager in charge of catering services, safety might mean maintaining the quality of food to avoid customer dissatisfaction or illness.
>
> In that case, how does he ensure that the food is of top quality? What sorts of control points and check points does he establish? How does he ensure that there is no deterioration in food quality in flight? Who checks the temperature of the refrigerators or the condition of the oven while the plane is in the air?
>
> Only when safety is translated into specific actions with specific control and check points established for each employee's job may safety be said to have been truly deployed as a policy. Policy deployment calls for everyone to interpret policy in the light of his own responsibilities and for everyone to work out criteria to check his success in carrying out the policy.

Imai's example is particularly relevant to the many organizations which state clearly in their publicity or policy statements that there will be no discrimination against social class, ethnicity, religion, sexuality, disability etc. The reality for customers or users of those organizations may be very different. The test is whether these statements are translated into specific policies and specific actions to ensure that this often genuine statement of intent actually happens.

For example, Cambridge University say in their prospectus that college admission tutors 'aim to make our selection [of prospective students] regardless of candidates' social, educational or personal backgrounds'. However if, as is widely believed, admission tutors give preference to students from schools which have previously sent students to that college or to those with a parent who attended that college, then there will be systematic discrimination. Policy statements on equal access need to be translated into the actual admissions policies, otherwise they are worthless.

Policy deployment

Policy deployment is a translation of the Japanese phrase *hoshin kanri* which has been used very successfully in that country. It is the process by which strategic plans are deployed, cascaded and implemented throughout the organization. It enables an organization to identify its key challenges, facilitating two-way communication, and provides a framework for decision making and prioritizing work. It brings the vision into reality and provides a way of educating staff about the aims of the organization and how to bring them about. Policy deployment is also important for staff. As Harr (2001) says, 'A factor, which should not be underestimated, is clear goal focus for the organisation. Staff want a sense of purpose in their work, a goal they can identify with. 90 per cent of staff motivation comes from clearly defined goals'.

A model for policy deployment in health and social care is illustrated in Figure 5.8. It begins with the organization's vision, values and mission statement. The mission statement is then translated into specific goals taking into account the needs of all stakeholders. Measures and targets are set and strategies to achieve these targets are designed. Finally, strategies are translated into operational policies to improve processes.

Clinical Governance is an example of policy deployment. Rather than simply exhorting staff to improve the quality of care (which would be an example of what Oakland calls 'goals without methods' (Oakland 1999)), clinical governance recognizes that more guidance is required on how this might be done. Referring to Figure 5.8, it involves looking at the needs of patients, staff and other stakeholders, together with relevant measures of performance. Targets are set and strategies developed to meet those targets. These strategies are then translated into process improvements.

Going beyond the mission statement: requirements for effective policy deployment

The following are essential if policy deployment is to work effectively (based on Ernst & Young Quality Improvement Consulting Group 1992).

- Top management is responsible for developing and communicating a vision, then building organization-wide commitment to its achievement.
- The vision is deployed through the development and execution of annual policy statements (plans).
- All levels of employees actively participate in generating a strategy and action plans to attain this vision.

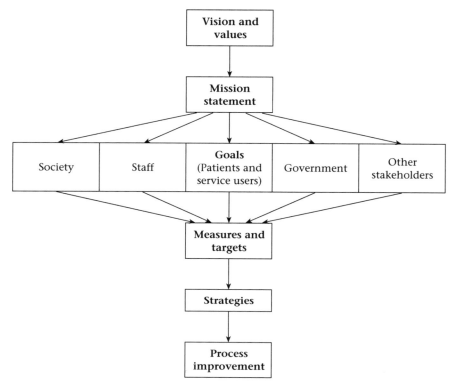

Figure 5.8 Policy deployment in health and social care

- At each level, progressively more detailed and concrete means to accomplish the annual plans are determined. The plans are hierarchical, cascading downward from top management's plans. There should be a clear link to common goals in activities throughout the organization.
- Each organizational level sets priorities to focus on areas needing significant improvement, and to concentrate on activities that are most closely related to the vision.
- Implementation responsibilities, timetables and progress measures are determined.
- Frequent evaluation, and modification based on feedback from regularly scheduled audits of the process, are provided.
- Plans and actions are developed based on analysis of the root causes of a problem, rather than only on the symptoms.
- Planning has a high degree of detail, including the anticipation of possible problems during implementation.
- Emphasis is on the improvement of the process, as opposed to a results-only orientation.

Policy deployment at Center Parcs

It is interesting to examine policy deployment in a service organization in the private sector committed to excellent service – Center Parcs All Season Holidays. Their mission statement is: 'To give our guests a truly unique short break holiday experience which far exceeds their expectations'. They realized however that they needed to give more guidance to their staff about how the mission could be carried out. Included with the mission statement are the following 'six basic goals':

- *Goal 1*: We will achieve this through our visionary approach to creative management.
- *Goal 2*: By continually striving for the highest standards of product possible.
- *Goal 3*: By having an approach to guest service that is second to none.
- *Goal 4*: By a positive approach to the genuine recognition of our own employees.
- *Goal 5*: Through a commitment to invest in the business and in the personal development of each and every individual in the organization.
- *Goal 6*: This will result in our guest returning, in satisfying our employees needs and ultimately in optimizing the profitability of our company, thus maintaining our position as market leader and securing our own future.

It may be noted that if we substitute 'user' or 'patient' for 'guest' and add something about access and equal opportunities, the first five goals could be relevant to many organizations in health and social care.

Policy deployment at Kingston upon Hull City Council

Some people in the public sector dislike the terms 'mission' and 'vision', but nevertheless recognize the need to provide a clear lead to its staff, users and other stakeholders. To conclude this chapter we look at the example of Hull City Council, who have what they call an 'over-arching' aim and four corporate aims (see Figure 5.9), together with a statement of their organizational values. These values are:

- The provision of quality, best value services, aspiring to top ten performance.
- Working in partnership with others to secure the economic, social and environmental well-being of our communities.
- The promotion of sustainability, equality of opportunity and equality of access.
- The development of the City Council's community leadership role.
- Open, responsive, accountable government, involving local people in transparent decision making.
- High standards of integrity in the conduct of the City Council's business, and in dealing with the public.

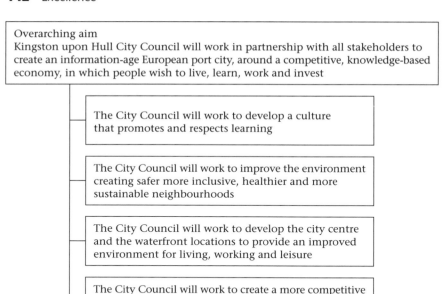

Figure 5.9   Policy deployment at Kingston upon Hull City Council

The above values are only the starting point. Hull have developed a number of key objectives for each of the corporate aims and for each key objective they have a position statement, a statement of key issues and a list of performance targets. These statements and values can give a clear lead to staff and also keep users informed. However it is also important that the organization delivers what it promises and that expectations are not raised unrealistically. Otherwise, as was noted in Chapter 2, users will be dissatisfied when their expectations are not met.

CHAPTER SIX

People development and involvement

It is somewhat patronizing and clichéd, but nevertheless true, to say that the success of all organizations in health and social care is achieved through people. Excellently written policy statements and standards, and carefully designed processes cannot deliver quality health and social care unless the needs of staff are recognized and met. People development and involvement are a vital part of the drive towards excellence. As the Cabinet Office's (1999) document *Assessing Excellence* says, 'you should always bear in mind that it is staff who must implement changes and must make the revised systems work. Leaders cannot change the performance of the organisation on their own. It is therefore essential to involve staff fully not only in the assessment process, but also in making the changes that stem from that assessment'.

Comments like the following are extremely common in organizations in all sectors of the economy: 'If that's what management wants, then that's what we'll do. But it would be much better if we did...' Whatever the organization, one thing is certain: the group the person belongs to will not be providing the best service they could. The expertise and experience of those doing the job has not been harnessed. Management have not asked them what they would do, nor have they listened to their views. Management have also not communicated the benefits of the method imposed to the staff involved. Because staff do not feel part of this decision, whatever the merits of the idea, quality is likely to suffer.

Other comments that can be heard every day in many organizations are: 'How can they expect me to improve quality when I have to use this clapped out old machine?'; 'Our quality has always been OK, it's the XYZ department they need to look at'; 'How can they expect me to do any more when I spend half my life in this downtrodden place?' It is clear from these three quotes that issues affecting staff have not been addressed. Morale and motivation is poor and again these people will be unlikely to provide a quality service. To achieve real quality improvement an organization has to address the issues as experienced by its staff. There must be a real commitment to them. If we want people to value the customer then it is important that they in turn feel valued and supported by the organization.

As an example, I remember visiting the city centre branch of my bank and happened to look over the reception desk and see a notice behind the counter saying, 'Smile, you are on reception'. However, what I also saw behind the counter was one very harassed member of staff on her own with a queue of customers. She was clearly unsupported and some distance away from other staff who could help her. Management must give their staff a reason to smile – particularly if they want that smile to be genuine. They need to ensure that reception is adequately staffed, that staff get adequate breaks and are given appropriate training. If the customer wants some information, is this easily available and not out of stock? Are there written down procedures to help deal with common problems? Are the people on reception involved in discussions about how best to treat customers with particular problems?

The importance of managing people can be seen from the success of Japanese manufacturing industry whose achievements in producing high quality products at low cost is well known. This is well expressed in the following quote from a Japanese executive of CBS/Sony some years ago:

> Lately we have been having a number of visitors from the United States and Europe who want to observe our latest technology in phonograph record making. They know that our records sound better, but once they step inside our factory they discover that we use the same technology, the same pressing machine and the same raw materials. Some visitors insist that we are using secret solutions and want to inspect our residue. Of course they do not find anything that they do not find in their residues at home. They look puzzled when I tell them that the difference in quality of sound comes from our people and not from our machines.

This statement summarises well the main reasons for the success of Japanese industries. While other factors are of course relevant, including the level of investment in the factory, of most importance are those addressed by the three Cs in Oakland's model of TQM (see Chapter 2), namely: commitment, culture and communication. Although the UK culture is very different to that of the Japanese, without proper attention to the three Cs no organization can deliver excellent service.

There are a number of requirements for effective people management (see Figure 6.1), each leading to improved performance. These are now considered in turn.

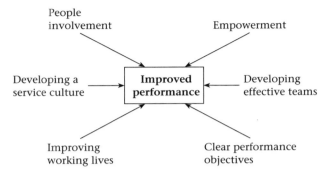

Figure 6.1 Requirements for effective people management

People involvement and empowerment

People involvement and empowerment are vital for delivering excellence and in creating the right environment for change. Indeed, Lesley Munro-Faure, Chief Executive of the European Forum for Teamwork, says that 'genuine involvement and empowerment is the most powerful change mechanism of all'.

People involvement, or employee involvement (EI) as it is sometimes known, aims to transform an organization's culture to utilize the creative energies of all employees for problem solving and for making improvements. With EI, the roles of employees at all levels within the organization are re-examined. The basic philosophy is that management should provide support for front-line employees, rather than just try to control them. Top managers must share and delegate some of the tasks which they previously kept to themselves. Rather than pretend to be 'in control', they should acknowledge that others have an important role to play in decisions that they previously made with minimum consultation. One of top management's new roles will be in setting up a quality steering committee or quality council to oversee EI activities.

Middle managers too have a different role to play. As front-line workers become more involved in decisions affecting their area of work, the traditional role of middle management becomes eroded and many feel threatened by the new situation. It is true that managers who are unable or unwilling to adopt more participative styles of management may be at risk, but in fact middle managers have several new roles. These include translating top management's vision, mission and strategy into their area of responsibility, providing feedback to top management and aligning top management's vision with the needs of staff in their area. Front-line employees generally accept the changes EI involves, though only if they perceive that managers genuinely want to involve them and listen to their needs.

Gufreda *et al.* (1992) give a number of advantages of EI over traditional management approaches:

- it replaces the adversarial 'us versus them' mentality with trust, cooperation and common goals;
- it helps develop individual capability by improving self-management and leadership skills, creating a sense of mission and fostering trust;
- it increases employee morale and commitment;
- it fosters creativity and innovation, the source of competitive advantage;
- it helps people understand quality principles and instils these into the corporate culture;
- it allows employees to solve problems at the source immediately;
- it improves quality and productivity.

The following quote from Philip Caldwell, the chief executive of Ford, shows the benefits of EI to individuals:

> The magic of employee involvement is that it allows individuals to discover their own potential – and to put that potential to work in more creative ways. A survey last year of more than 750 EI participants at seven facilities found that a full 82% felt they had a chance to accomplish something worthwhile, compared with only 27% before EI was initiated. People develop in themselves pride in workmanship, self-respect, self-reliance and a heightened sense of responsibility.
>
> (Caldwell 1984)

Empowerment

Empowerment goes beyond EI. Empowered employees make decisions in their area themselves and are responsible for their outcomes. The benefits to the organization can be summed up by the following quote from Mike Perides of the British Quality Foundation: 'When you hire a pair of hands, you get a brain free. You need to tap into that creativity and innovation potential'. This can be illustrated by considering a receptionist at a hotel when a guest arrives on a Sunday morning with a particular problem that needs resolving that morning. The receptionist can reply, 'Sorry, I need to talk to my manager but she is not back until Monday', or receptionists can be empowered by the manager to make certain decisions themselves to address the guest's concerns without needing to refer to the manager. In the first case, providing service quality is not a possibility. While most hotels adopt the former model (in which case there is no possibility of 'delighting the customer'), Ritz-Carlton Hotels is one group who *do* authorize staff to spend up to a given amount in responding to a guest's problems.

Empowering individuals is a major step. It is important to be clear about the limits of their responsibility and authority. Jan Carlzon (1987) puts this very clearly:

You must provide a framework in which people can act. For example, we have said that our first priority is safety, second is punctuality and third is other services. So, if you risk flight safety by leaving on time, you have acted outside the framework of your authority. The same is true if you don't leave on time because you are missing two catering boxes of meat. That's what I mean by a framework, you give people a framework, and within that framework you let people act.

'Empowerment is a state of mind', say Bowen and Lawler (1994). An employee with an empowered state of mind, they continue:

experiences feelings of (1) control over how the job shall be performed; (2) awareness of the context in which the work is performed and where it fits in the 'big picture'; (3) accountability for personal work output; (4) shared responsibility for unit and organisational performance; and (5) equity in the distribution of rewards based on individual and collective performance.

For empowerment to work effectively, there needs to be mutual trust between senior managers and staff. As Juran (1989) says, 'The managers must trust the workforce enough to be willing to make the delegation, and the workforce must have enough confidence in the managers to be willing to accept that responsibility'. Also important for empowerment to work is for employees to have access to information on the performance of their department or organization. They also need to be given appropriate training and development to help them adjust to changed methods of working.

Developing effective teams

Teamwork is an important part of TQM and business excellence. Senge (1992) states that high performing successful teams have one thing in common: they all have a clear vision and purpose. He suggests that when a team has a 'shared vision' then they start to talk about 'our team' and 'our company' rather than 'the company'.

Developing effective teams is an important part of being a good manager or leader. A useful model in this context is that by Adair (1987) illustrated in Figure 6.2. A team leader needs to be aware of three different types of need: those of the task, those of the team and those of individuals. For the task, clear achievable targets and standards of performance are needed, while team needs include a supportive climate and a common sense of purpose and identity. Individuals need to be accepted and valued both by the leader and by the team, and to have scope for personal growth and development.

The requirements of a good football manager illustrate very well the importance of addressing all three aspects. To be successful, the manager has

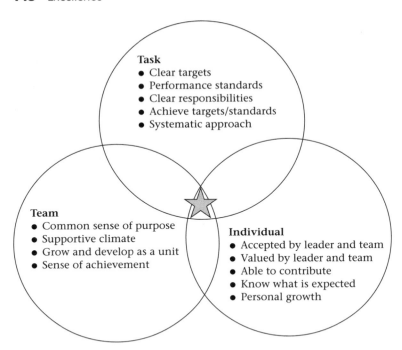

Figure 6.2 Adair's model, based on Oakland (1999: 160)

to deliver results – trophies, promotion to the next division, or avoiding relegation – but they cannot do this without welding individuals into a team, or working with individual players to develop their skills.

The team leader or facilitator needs to concentrate on the small area where the three circles overlap (marked with a star), and aim to satisfy all three sets of needs – achieving the task, building the team and satisfying individuals. Some team leaders are good at creating team spirit, but do not focus sufficiently on the task or on individuals. Others might focus exclusively on the task, and indeed achieve short-term successes. For sustained excellence, however, all three areas need to be addressed.

Figure 6.3 shows the individual functions that the team leader has to perform to meet each of the three areas. The everyday example of allocating work to individuals in a social care team shows the difficulties in addressing all three aspects simultaneously. For example, if a difficult case needs to be allocated to a social worker, the manager needs to choose someone with the necessary expertise to make sure the task gets done efficiently, but without upsetting others who may feel they could do the task, thereby adversely affecting the team culture. Also, the manager needs to ensure that the person chosen feels valued and not overloaded.

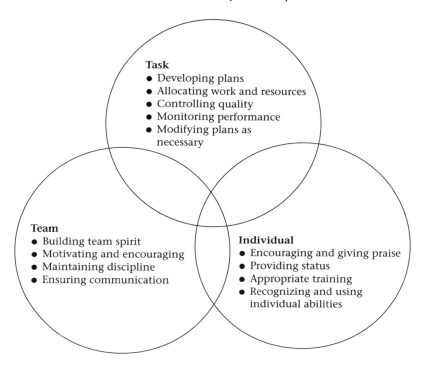

Figure 6.3 Functions of an effective team leader

Teams for quality improvement

There are a great many types of team in different organizations. These include:

- *Operational teams*: who perform a given function or process together, but are not given overall responsibility. These are of course very common in both health and social care.
- *Quality circles*: teams of workers and supervisors that meet regularly to address quality-related problems.
- *Quality improvement teams*: teams who gather to tackle a specific problem and then disband.
- *Self-managed teams*: who work as a team and are responsible for producing a well-defined product or service.
- *Management teams*: consisting mainly of managers from various functions.
- *Virtual teams*: these communicate by computer, take turns as leader and jump in or out as necessary.

Quality circles, quality improvement teams and self-managed teams are now discussed in more detail.

Quality circles

Quality circles are groups of between 3 and 12 employees who do the same or similar work, voluntarily meeting regularly for about one hour per week in paid time. They are led by a trained leader and discuss and solve work-related problems. These problems are chosen by the group itself and the solutions are presented to management. In many cases the solutions are implemented and controlled by circle members. There is usually a link between the circle leader and a quality circle steering committee, which includes senior managers, to give circles the support they need.

Typically a quality circle will begin by drawing up a list of possible topics for consideration by brainstorming techniques. The circle will then select the main problems they wish to consider, identify the main causes of the problems and put mechanisms in place to get feedback on the causes of these particular problems in the future.

The group might again use brainstorming to come up with a list of possible solutions, discuss them and establish which ones they wish to adopt. These solutions are then presented to management and, provided they have no objection, will be implemented by the group which then selects the next problem or problems to tackle.

There are a number of success criteria for quality circles to work effectively (based on Philips 1986):

• Membership of a circle should be entirely voluntary, and care taken in training circle leaders to create an environment where no one feels shy, and everyone can participate to the full.
• Attention should be given to identifying the 'right' problem for the circle to look at. It has to be 'right' in the sense that it motivates the individuals concerned; 'right' in that it is within the competence of the group to solve it; and 'right' in the sense that there is a chance that management will actually implement the solution offered.
• Support from other people within the organization is vital. This includes the involvement of all departmental personnel, whether circle members or not, and support from specialists (e.g. purchasing, engineering, and organization and efficiency).
• Support from top management is essential. How senior managers react to circle suggestions, and how they feed back their decisions with regard to these suggestions, is critical for continued motivation.
• Support from the departmental manager is also important. These managers are in a very difficult position. They must be supportive without being dominant.

Quality circles at Ash Grove residential home

When staff at Ash Grove residential home in Wakefield decided to form a quality action group to help improve services at the home, they were initially rather anxious that they would raise expectations which they could not meet. However, when they went ahead they discovered that it was the day-to-day issues which were more important to residents.

They began by asking residents what aspects of their care were most important to them and what things they liked and disliked. One issue raised was that when they wanted things from the shops, they were not then able to choose for themselves. Staff were willing to shop for them (e.g. for birthday cards) but the choice was limited.

Staff also found that they spent a great deal of time running off to the shops when they felt they could be giving more care to the residents. What residents and staff came up with was the idea of a shopping trolley containing a number of items that residents regularly requested.

Staff consulted residents about what should be on the trolley and ran a quiz to select the trolley's name ('AG Homestore' was the winning entry). Birthday cards, sweets, crisps, cigarettes, stockings and other personal items such as hairgrips were decided on. For birthday cards, for example, a range was kept in stock with the designs residents liked. They also got together to decide how many of each item they should buy and set up systems to identify what was low on stock and which items were nearing their sell-by date. Standards were set up – for example, that the trolley service was available between 10 and 11 a.m. and between 3 and 4 p.m. They also set up a system to monitor whether the standards were being achieved.

The key benefits of this scheme were:

- it got residents involved and interested;
- it got staff working together with each other, and with residents, on a project;
- it increased choice for residents;
- it saved time, enabling better care of residents;
- it helped develop staff understanding of quality processes;
- it created a sense of achievement for all involved, to encourage continuous quality improvement.

Quality improvement teams

Quality improvement teams, or cross-functional teams as they are sometimes called, are groups of people brought together by management to examine a particular problem, such as improving discharge procedures or reducing waiting lists at a hospital. These are particularly common in health care: for example, taskforces and Clinical Governance teams. They typically include people from different professional groups and backgrounds and will disband once the project has been completed.

To be effective such a group will need a wide remit covering anything that is relevant to the problem being tackled and must have the authority and backing of senior managers.

Self-managed teams

Many organizations, although mostly in the private sector, have adopted the self-managed team concept, which increases both participation and empowerment. Self-managed teams involve a highly trained group of employees (between 6 and 18 people) fully responsible for turning out a well-defined segment of finished work. This could be a final product like a ball bearing, or a service like a fully-processed insurance claim. One of the early pioneers of this approach was Volvo in Sweden. Suitable candidates in health and social care could be a pharmacy, a laboratory or a particular scheme for providing respite care.

Self-managed teams have a number of characteristics (based on Wellins *et al.* 1991):

- they are empowered to take on various management and leadership functions;
- they plan, control and improve their own work processes;
- they set their own goals and inspect their own work;
- they take responsibility for the quality of their products and services.

Many teams in health and social care exhibit some characteristics of self-managed teams, but relatively few can be regarded as self-managed in the sense given above.

Clear performance objectives

Another vital part of improving employee performance is effective performance management. Performance management has a bad name in some areas, but this is mainly where it has been implemented poorly. Effective performance management of staff involves giving clear objectives showing what is expected of them, ensuring that they are given appropriate resources, training and development to fulfil those objectives, two-way communication so that they can feed information and their experiences back to senior managers, and appropriate recognition of their efforts.

The NHS in Scotland identifies five aspects of motivating and developing employees (Audit Scotland 2001):

- *Setting objectives.* Setting out clearly what employees are expected to do is a fundamental part of managing performance. As the Audit Commission (1997) says, 'If people are clear about what they should be doing, and know how their job contributes to the larger picture, they tend to be more committed: the result is higher productivity and better quality services'. Objectives for staff should be clearly linked to those at a departmental and organizational level. They also need to be specific, measurable, action-oriented, realistic, and have timescales for action (SMART).

- *Assessing development needs.* Assessing training and development needs to ensure employees improve their ability to reach the expected standard of performance. Development needs can be met in a number of ways including work shadowing, mentoring, coaching and guidance, study for professional qualifications, on-the-job training and giving staff new responsibilities. Development needs to be linked to the goals of the organization. For example, if the aim is to improve patient care, then appropriate training and development to help achieve this will be needed. Mike Wistow, Head of Corporate Performance Management at Hull City Council, emphasizes the significance of this, saying that 'staff training and development requires investment and is the single most important factor in actually improving quality and developing a continuous improvement culture'.
- *Making it happen.* Improving communication between senior managers, line managers and staff not only to inform them but also to ensure that senior leaders get to know the expectations and ideas of their staff. Morale, motivation, frustration, enthusiasm and commitment all affect performance and it is vital to listen to and act on employees' views and suggestions. The following two quotes from George Mackay of BT are useful here: 'Communication can be like a damp-proof course. Nothing goes up and nothing comes down' and 'We each have two ears and one mouth. Used in that proportion we'll be OK'.
- *Review.* Having set objectives for individual employees, it is important to review them regularly so that employees feel recognized for their achievement and can identify areas where performance can improve. It is also important to monitor whether development needs identified previously have actually happened, while another aspect of the review is to make sure that the performance measures given are both fair and realistic.
- *Doing better.* The aim of this phase is to identify areas for improvement in the performance of individual employees. In order to improve performance, people need to be clear about what they should do, have the skills and experience required, know how well they have performed and how they could do better. Discussions on performance need to feed into the first two stages. While staff should be given positive feedback and encouragement on their achievements, they also need a clear mechanism for improving performance.

As mentioned at the start of this section, it is also important to ensure that staff are given appropriate resources, training, development and support to achieve the objectives set. Indeed, it is lack of attention to these factors that has sometimes given performance management a bad name. This is recognized by the Working Together programme, which is part of the NHS Human Resources Performance Management Framework and addresses the issue of improving human resource management standards within the NHS. One of the strategic aims of this initiative is 'to ensure that we have a quality workforce, in the right numbers, with the right skills and diversity, organised in the right way, to deliver the Government's service objectives for health and social care' (Department of Health 1998b). To achieve these aims, the Working Together programme recognizes the need for a strong system of underpinning values – fairness and equality, flexibility, efficiency and partnership working – a commitment to working together on a common agenda for action, clear measures of progress and a proper system for review and evaluation.

Improving working lives

Another key aspect of getting the best out of people is a recognition that improving the working lives of staff both helps to deliver better care and also reduce costs through improved recruitment and retention. This is explicitly recognized by the Improving Working Lives Initiative, which is part of the NHS Human Resources Performance Management Framework. There are a number of aspects to this initiative:

- improving human resource management practices, leading to improvements in the quality of working lives for staff;
- commitment to more flexible, supportive, family friendly and culturally sensitive ways of working and training;
- working with staff to develop a range of more flexible working practices that balance the needs of patients and services with the needs of staff;
- valuing and supporting staff and ensuring they are treated with dignity and respect;
- providing personal and professional development and training opportunities that are accessible and open to all staff irrespective of their working patterns;
- enabling staff to manage a healthy balance between work and their commitments outside work, including accessible, affordable and good quality child care;
- ensuring that human resource policies are applied fairly to all staff regardless of age, ethnicity, gender, staff group or working patterns.

Another aspect which should be addressed is the physical environment in which staff work. Large numbers of staff in social care and health work in an environment which is not conducive to them feeling valued. This too needs urgent attention.

Developing a service culture

Another important aspect of people development is to facilitate staff moving to a culture of putting patients and users at the heart of services. Most employees in health and social care interact with service users and there must be both commitment and example from senior managers and clinicians to a service culture, and appropriate training and development in relating to service users. As Sir Donald Irvine, past president of the General Medical Council, puts it: 'today we are consumers in a service-minded world where the public, not the providers, expect to call the shots'.

In particular, staff need to reassure users that they see services from their viewpoint and take responsibility for finding a solution to problems which satisfies the user. They need to respect users as individuals, listen to them and deal with them promptly and courteously. Finally staff need to show that they can be trusted and care about the services users receive. As one service user, quoted in *Putting the Person First* (National Institute for Social Work 2001), put it: 'A lot of it is about attitude. If you get the right attitude everything else will follow'. This is backed up by studies reported by Triseliotis *et al.* (1995) which indicate that the following characteristics are the qualities that families and foster carers want from their social workers:

Families want social workers who are purposeful, genuine, consistent, open and honest, trustworthy, businesslike, take tasks seriously and are participative.

Foster carers want social workers who offer recognition, praise and reassurance, build rapport and are energetic, knowledgeable and committed.

The area of trust is particularly relevant. The following are some guidelines to help staff exude trust (Hopson and Scally 1991):

- be open and honest about themselves;
- take responsibility;
- admit mistakes and shortcomings;
- keep promises;
- be consistent;
- be prepared to put themselves out.

Another important aspect of a service culture, according to Hopson and Scally (1991), is to make sure that proper attention is given to service users during the first four and the last two minutes of any encounter. The statement 'first impressions count' is getting a bit hackneyed but is nevertheless as true as ever. People rapidly assess how important they are (or are not) in the eyes of the other person and how much the other person cares, is enthusiastic, willing to help or otherwise. Rapport not built in the first four minutes is difficult to establish later. Another particularly important time is the last two minutes of an encounter. These last two minutes can be utilized to avoid giving a user the feeling that they have now been 'processed' and that the organization is no longer interested in them. Instead, there is an opportunity to create a feeling of warmth which creates a good lasting impression.

Although particular attention is needed at these times, all time spent with a service user or carer affects their impressions of the service and the organization. People are often insecure and anxious when they arrive at a given facility, particularly if it is their first encounter with that organization. Patients and service users may not know what is expected of them or what will happen to them. If they feel uncared for at the start, that impression may remain.

Training front-line staff in customer care is an important part of developing a service culture. They will learn skills such as using the person's name, listening to them, being empathetic, greeting them with enthusiasm, avoiding negative comments and the appearance of being rushed. Also important is assessing what kind of help people want – for example, to be left alone, to be approached, to be chatted to or to be direct with. The importance of staff developing these skills can be seen from this quote taken from the Wiltshire Users' Network (Harding and Beresford 1996): 'So often it is the style of the way services are delivered, rather than the service itself, which produces a quality service. The home carer who gets you up in the morning can do this in an empowering way which enables you to face the effort of the day positively, or in a way which means you are dressed and ready but not psychologically ready'.

There are a great variety of service users in the public sector, some of whom will be uncooperative and even hostile. However, even in these situations it is important for staff to see things from the viewpoint of the service user. Giving patients and families bad news is one such situation, while an example from housing is a member of staff who has been asked to collect rent arrears. Discussing the latter on a customer care course, staff from Birmingham City Council decided that a customer care approach should centre on finding out why the tenant was unable to pay, rather than seeing the task of collecting the rent as all-important. In social care, staff frequently have to inform people that they have not been approved as prospective adopters or that their child will be taken into care. Good practice here is for staff to be open and honest about why the decision was made, giving clear information and explaining why they believe this to be in the best interests of the children concerned.

Twelve steps to a service culture

To conclude this chapter, the following 12 steps to a service culture, adapted from Hopson and Scally (1991), illustrate that developing a service culture involves much more than putting staff on customer care courses. It must be an integral part of the way the organization operates.

Step 1: Decide on your key mission and core values. Identify the main purpose of your department or unit. This should define who you are providing a service for and reflect the needs of relevant stakeholders and your core values.

Step 2: Know your service users and other stakeholders. Talk to your patients, carers, service users and other stakeholders. Find out their requirements and expectations. Consider how well you currently meet their expectations and identify, with service users where possible, ways of better meeting their needs. Also, remember to treat service users as individuals and not to let them think they are being processed. As a respondent to a recent British Airways customer survey said: 'Treat us as people, as individuals, don't just process us!'

Step 3: Create your vision. Like your statement of your core business, the statement of the vision of your organization (see Chapter 5) gives a lead to your staff and, hopefully, the right message to service users.

Step 4: Define your moments of truth. Moments of truth (see Chapter 1) are those encounters between users and your organization that will make the biggest difference to how they perceive the service they have received. Make sure that processes are designed to ensure that these moments of truth provide the best possible service. In health and social care do not underestimate the difference you can make in a single short interaction.

Step 5: Give good service to one another. The quality of service that impacts on patients and service users begins with the quality of service that staff give each other. This includes different staff within your organization and other partners and stakeholders. Leadership and support from management, together with a commitment to partnership working, are important here.

Step 6: Create the service user experience. Service excellence does not happen by chance. It has to be carefully planned. In addition to designing the core service, with the help of users stakeholders and partners, managers need to ensure that staff have the relevant skills and training, both in the technical nature of the job and in how they interact with service users. As Sir Donald Irvine says: 'Doctors must be taught to be as competent in interpersonal skills as they are in more traditional clinical skills'. In creating the service user experience, staff also need to consider whether users and patients are given the information they need. Are they told what is likely to happen, are they greeted on arrival, do they feel listened to or do they feel they are being processed? Do staff demonstrate a positive attitude and give clear messages?

Step 7: Profit from complaints. Complaints are a vital source of information for any organization. While the vast majority of dissatisfied users do not complain, the information obtained from those that do can be very illuminating. Encouraging users to provide feedback on their experiences – and acting on that feedback – will enable you to offer an even better service.

Step 8: Stay close to your service users and other stakeholders. Involve your service users and other stakeholders when developing your plans for the service, reassuring them and helping them to understand what to expect.

Step 9: Design and implement the service programme. This is the decisive step that some managers find difficult. It is moving from making a series of improvements in service quality to a well-defined service improvement programme providing a lead and encompassing all the different aspects of quality. One of the main aims of this book is to assist managers in achieving this.

Step 10: Set performance standards and measures. Setting (and monitoring) performance standards and measures is an important vehicle for ensuring that the various aspects of service quality important to users and carers are actually delivered.

Step 11: Recognize and reward service excellence. In many cases staff who provide excellent service get direct feedback and recognition from users and patients. This can be the best feedback of all, but if you want your staff to continue to give real service to users, then the organization has to systematically recognize that this has been done and give some recognition and reward to the individual concerned. Make sure that service factors are considered alongside other factors when considering staff for promotion, for example.

Step 12: Develop the service programme. This is similar to Crosby's 'do it all over again' (see Chapter 2). You have made a good start by following the first 11 steps – now is the time to reflect on what you have done and develop the next stage of the programme. The Excellence Model is a good guide to have with you here.

CHAPTER seven

Partnerships and user involvement

Developing partnerships has been recognized as an essential part of many government initiatives including Best Value, the NHS Plan, Quality Protects and Clinical Governance. Effective partnerships are needed with other departments within the same organization, between different agencies or Trusts, between GPs and hospitals, between health, social care, housing and education, and with the voluntary sector. In practice, however, partnership working in health and social care is often limited to occasional meetings of people from different agencies.

The importance of user involvement in health and social care is also identified in many government initiatives and research projects. This is considered later in this chapter (see p. 165).

Managing quality across organizational boundaries

Perhaps more than any other profession, health and social care staff work across organizational and professional boundaries all the time. As a result, a lot of experience and good practice is built up over the years. However, while all groups have a common aim to deliver services to improve life for patients and service users, different agencies and professions have different cultures, priorities, working methods and even language. The need for cooperation is illustrated by an example a few years ago in which South Yorkshire Police, the probation service and the social services department were each asked to name the top ten people in Sheffield that they were worried about. Nine families appeared on all three lists, but there was at the time little cooperation between the three services.

Managing quality across organizational boundaries is vital for a quality service. A high proportion of patients and service users come into regular contact with a variety of professionals both within health and social services and in other organizations. This has many implications for quality. Mental health workers, for example, are unlikely to get a high rating for their service by users whose housing needs are not met, whatever the level of service provided. Similarly, housing staff will not get a good rating if their clients' mental health needs are not properly met. To get a high rating for quality, mental health and housing workers need to work together in an effective partnership to ensure that the users' mental health and housing needs are both met. This example emphasizes the importance of partnership working between health and social care and other agencies. It is also one of the key areas addressed by the Best Value initiative.

Another area where partnership working is essential is in addressing drug misuse. This clearly cannot be tackled without social services, the NHS, the police, the probation service, housing, education, the voluntary sector and private industry (e.g. pubs and clubs) all working together and understanding each other's role. Discharging older people from hospital is another area in which there is a potential for conflict between different professionals – in this case between social workers, nurses, clinicians and occupational therapists. The Scottish Office Social Work Services Group (1998) concluded that 'Hospital discharge is too frequently characterised by clashing professional perspectives. The limited involvement of the housing and voluntary sector is a cause for concern. There is also some element of duplication of effort, particularly between occupational therapy and social work assessments'.

The following example looks at a typical situation where roles conflict or are unclear. All names have of course been changed.

Deborah is a single mother with a 10-year-old son, a new baby and Andrew, who is 2 and suffers from severe uncontrolled epilepsy. Four different professionals regularly visit the family at home:

- Jane, a social worker for children with disabilities who is based at the general hospital;
- Brian, a community nurse based at a community health centre;
- Surita, a health visitor based at Deborah's GP; and
- Ginny, a portage worker, responsible for pre-nursery education for children with special needs, from the council's education department.

In addition, Deborah and Andrew regularly see the consultant at the hospital, ward staff, physiotherapists and occupational therapists.

Deborah is nervous about taking Andrew out of the home, partly because she is embarrassed at people's reaction when he fits, and in particular because she has to administer emergency rectal medication if he fits for more than five minutes. As a result Andrew has very little contact with other toddlers and this has increased his, and Deborah's, isolation. The professionals involved believe that the best policy might be for someone to accompany her to a local mother and toddlers group.

But who should it be? Should it be Surita, who knows the local area best? Should it be Ginny, who visits Deborah most often and possibly has the closest relationship with her? Should it be Brian, who knows most about administering the medication? Or should it be Jane, who has responsibilities not just for Andrew but also for Deborah's well-being and that of the rest of the family?

Such a situation, where the roles of professionals overlap and are unclear, is very common. Often there is no easy way to resolve these dilemmas and if people are not careful considerable time (offering no value to either Deborah or Andrew) can be spent in deciding who should do what. In this case, the problem could of course be resolved by asking Deborah who she would like to go with. After all, it is the needs of the patients and service users, not the professionals, which are paramount. However, the point is that relationships are not clear and each professional may not understand the role and responsibilities of the others.

One example of partnership working is the Working Together Better project in Leeds, which brought together staff from Leeds health authority and Leeds social services concerned with primary health care. This project aimed to improve communication between GP practices, primary health care staff and social services. This included lunchtime workshops (light lunch provided) where staff could come together and explore their roles and expectations of others. These workshops enabled different groups to see things from the perspective of others. Bronwen Holden, project coordinator, gives the following examples:

> Social workers will say the primary care team don't understand the referral process and expect them to act immediately. The primary care team will say they have difficulties contacting the duty team. GPs will say social workers complain that the GPs don't attend case conferences, but more often than not these meetings are held during surgery hours. By mixing up the groups, they begin to develop a better understanding of each other's situations and start to consider ways of improving communications. Even if some issues can't be resolved, then the fact that people have met face to face helps them to accept the differences in working cultures.
>
> (Bond 1998: 30–1)

Partnerships in intermediate care

Partnership working has been facilitated by the 1999 Health Act which allows health and social care agencies to pool funding to commission services. An example of this is in Sheffield where a partnership was formed between the four primary care groups in the city, two hospital trusts, a community health trust and the city council's social services department.

The partnership operates a community assessment and integrated care scheme which involves using four multi-disciplinary teams attached to each of the primary care groups to assess and meet the care needs of older people in their own homes. The teams each consist of a social worker, a physiotherapist, an occupational therapist, a therapy assistant and an administrative officer. The aim is to provide care for people who would otherwise have to be admitted to hospital as an emergency, but could remain at home were suitable support available. These include people who have suffered a fall or have chest or urinary infections. In addition to providing care closer to home, the partnership has a number of other objectives: improving the responsiveness of services, promoting independent living, increased choice for users and carers, reducing avoidable hospital stays and delaying entry into long-term care.

The teams assess the needs of the patient and then arrange for appropriate nursing and other support services and equipment to be provided at home. GPs can make a referral to them at any time, day or night, seven days a week, for an immediate assessment and the arrangement of appropriate services. They provide social and nursing care support and intensive home nursing. Barbara Nicholas, who is programme manager for intermediate care, said that most people prefer to be supported at home, provided they get the care they need: 'It is about giving people appropriate care. But it has the added benefit that it releases hospital beds for people whose needs are greater' (Midgley 2001).

The partnership also provides rehabilitation and resource centres in each of the primary care group areas. These are residential homes run by the local authority that have earmarked 26 beds for short-term care, rehabilitation and recuperation. Most are for patients who have been discharged from hospital but who are not yet ready to return home. The community assessment teams are based at these centres and nursing care is provided by intermediate care liaison nurses based at the two hospitals.

As an example of how the scheme works in practice, an 87-year-old woman with bad arthritis had been living independently in her own home with support from her family, but one day found that she could not get out of bed. Her GP, diagnosing a bad back, then called the local community assessment and integrated care team. An assessor arrived within two hours and concluded that the woman was at risk of falling and injuring herself. However, instead of suggesting hospital or admission to a care home, the assessor and his colleagues arranged immediately for a rapid response home care service to start visiting three times a day. This was followed by a physiotherapist's assessment, which led to regular therapy, and an occupational therapist who organized mobility aids and a pendant alarm (George 2001).

North East Derbyshire Community Mental Health Service

North East Derbyshire Community Mental Health Service has two main examples of working across organizational boundaries. First, the service is staffed jointly by health and social services under a single mental health services manager. This has successfully reduced the overlap and communication difficulties of working in separate departments under different bosses. Second, since access to a range of good quality accommodation is an essential component of community care for people with a mental illness, collaborative working arrangements have been established between housing and mental health services. Close links are also maintained with the local branch of the National Schizophrenia Fellowship.

At the core of the Mental Health Service are the care plan coordinators, who are experienced in mental health work and have an up-to-date knowledge of current health and social care provision. Whether employed by health or social services, they work across the boundaries and provide a single point of contact for the user. This reduces duplication of effort for the benefit of users, the team and the service as a whole and has resulted in improved relations between the agencies and greater ease and efficiency in organizing care packages.

The collaboration with housing staff has involved developing a protocol based on 'designated points of access'; one within the housing department and one within mental health services. This sets down the different ways housing staff who identify a possible mental health issue should approach mental health services, depending on the perceived urgency and how the mental health services should respond to that referral. In addition, since all care plans (and in particular discharge plans) need to ensure that a person's accommodation needs are met appropriately, the protocol also makes clear how mental health staff should contact housing services, again depending on the level of urgency, and how housing services should respond. Finally, arrangements are in place for resolving particular difficulties or disagreements between staff in different agencies.

Andrew Milroy, community social services manager for North East Derbyshire, gives this advice to others who are considering the development of collaborative working:

- Develop vision, belief and confidence.
- Obtain a clear understanding and agreement of what needs doing.
- Develop practical, understandable and realistic plans involving all relevant agencies.
- Leadership – especially by senior managers. It has never been more important to achieve the closest possible collaboration between public services and this requires real commitment to practical partnerships demonstrated from the top down.
- Be a heretic – be intolerant of people shoring up traditional boundaries which act as obstacles to the effective coordination of services.
- Put the local people who will use the service at the centre of all planning and create opportunities for people to be involved in the management and organization of the services they will use.

Principles of partnership working

Partnership working needs to exist at both macro and micro levels. The macro level refers to partnerships between organizations or agencies. These include partnerships between different agencies, departments or Trusts within health or social care, and those between organizations in different sectors such as health, social care, education, housing and the independent sector. Partnerships at the micro level are those between different professional groups (both in health and social care), between primary and secondary care, between local authorities and the voluntary sector, and also between NHS Trusts.

There are a number of barriers to partnership working that need to be addressed for partnerships to be effective. They include:

- lack of understanding of the roles and functions of other professions;
- not being aware of the different positions people have in other organizations and their ability to implement change (job titles can be misleading!);
- lack of understanding of the systems, procedures and regulations in different organizations;
- differences in ideology (e.g. between doctors and therapists, between health and social care and between the voluntary sector and other bodies).

The Nuffield Institute for Health, in association with NHS Executive Trent, have identified six partnership principles for effective partnership working (Hardy *et al.* 2000):

- *Recognize and accept the need for partnership.* This involves identifying the main partnership arrangements that have gone on in recent years and the main successes and barriers. It also involves recognition that an individual organization cannot achieve all its goals without working in partnerships.
- *Develop clarity and realism of purpose.* Partnerships need to be built on a shared vision, shared values and agreed service principles. If there are differences in perspective, these will need to be acknowledged. Realistic joint objectives should be identified, and expressed as outcomes for users. Areas where there is early partnership success should also be identified.
- *Ensure commitment and ownership.* There must be a clear commitment to partnership working both from senior staff in each organization and from those working at the operational level. Those with networking skills should be recognized and given positive encouragement.
- *Develop and maintain trust.* All partners must be accorded equal status, irrespective of the level of resources available. This is particularly true of partnerships with voluntary organizations. Trust built up within partnerships needs to be protected from any mistrust that develops in parent organizations.
- *Create robust and clear partnership working arrangements.* This principle involves transparency in the financial (and non-financial) resources each partner brings to the partnership. It should be clear what are each partner's

Table 7.1 Organizations people need to contact when moving house

Government	Social	Business	Industry
Land registry	GP	Estate agent	Gas
Planning department	Hospital	Solicitor	Electricity
Council	Dentist	Bank	Water
Electoral register	Internet	Insurance	Telephone
TV licence	Clubs/societies	Removals	Employer
Inland revenue			
Schools			

areas of responsibility and to whom they are accountable. The partnership's prime focus should be on process and outcomes, not structure and inputs.

• *Monitor, measure and learn.* Partnerships should have clear success criteria in terms of service goals and the partnership itself. Both of these elements should be monitored regularly and this feedback should be used to review the way the partnership operates, and its objectives. Finally, publicize successes!

Bob-Allen Turl of TNT, who is the chief executive of The Partnership Programme, in illustrating the need for better partnership working, suggests that people consider the different organizations they have to contact when moving house. A typical list is shown in Table 7.1. Turl points out that the only organizations in the list who talk to each other are the bank, the estate agent and the solicitor. The person moving has to deal with everyone else! This lack of partnership working between different organizations is one of the reasons that moving house is so stressful. Organizations in health and social care similarly should ask themselves the following questions: which groups of people and different organizations do their service users deal with; which of these groups does their department or organization talk to; and how can they develop partnerships to help ease users' path through the system?

User involvement

User involvement is a key area of both social care and health. For social care, Beresford (2000) puts it strongly: 'Not involving users is incompatible with the central aims of social work', while a key objective of Quality Protects is the 'participation of children, young people and their families in the planning and delivery of services and in decisions about their everyday lives' (Department of Health 1998d). In health services the Department of Health (1998a) states that 'Effective involvement of patients and carers is essential to ensuring that everyone is fully engaged in the drive for quality, and that this focuses on what really matters'. User involvement is also considered vital for Clinical Governance.

Involving users is invaluable to the organization to help it provide user-responsive services, but it also has other benefits for users. For children and young people for example, there are a number of benefits to participation (McNeish 1999):

- increased self-esteem, in turn affecting physical and mental well-being;
- greater feeling of control of their lives and welfare;
- likely to provide access to necessary life skills and information;
- likely to cause carers to be more assertive with services, so services become more responsive;
- beneficial for achieving other outcomes, provided that users are involved in defining these outcomes.

There are a variety of forms of user involvement:

- *User friendly.* This involves some representation, but fairly minimal. Staff are clearly the experts and in control. An example would be asking people in a residential home what colour they would like the carpets or what food they would like. There is no real consultation on the core service or how it is provided.
- *User centred.* Here there is more representation and users are asked their opinion about the whole range of services. Service users may be well represented in a management group, but all the key decisions on resources, staffing etc. are taken by the management.
- *User controlled.* This arrangement is set up and run by users and funded independently. An example might be a drop-in centre or a self-help group.

For effective user involvement in planning decisions, users need to be involved at two different levels: at senior management level where decisions are taken about the future of services, and 'on the ground' with staff and first-line managers of specific services. In the NHS, the proposals for an independent patients' forum in each NHS Trust with the power to monitor, review and inspect all aspects of local health services from the patient's perspective are intended to address patient involvement at the strategic level. Similarly, the new Patient Advice and Liaison Services (PALS) are intended, according to Health Secretary Alan Milburn, to have 'the knowledge and clout to sort out problems' for patients. Whether the PALS will prove effective will depend on whether they are fully resourced and have the knowledge, time and power to make a difference. They also need to be visible and accessible to people of all cultures and to all parts of the health care system. However, there is a danger that this might replicate the experiences of some manufacturing companies where staff felt that quality was the responsibility of the quality department rather than the role of everyone in the company. PALS must not be seen as the policemen and policewomen of quality. Quality, and user involvement, must be seen as everyone's responsibility if services are to meet the NHS Plan's core principle to 'shape its services around the needs and preferences of individual patients, their families and their carers' (National Health Service 2000).

The guidance from the Department of Health (1999a) on patient and public participation in Clinical Governance does address these issues. They recommend that NHS organizations should include user representatives on Clinical Governance committees or groups, should involve users in quality improvement programmes (e.g. in all stages of the clinical audit process) and should provide training for both NHS professionals and users on effective patient and public involvement. The last point is very important. The ability to involve users effectively is a skill. If user involvement is not thought through or handled poorly, staff may feel they have not learned very much while users may feel it is just a 'talking shop' and vote with their feet.

Some very useful findings come from a study on the involvement of children, young people and their families in the planning of children's services reported by Wiffen (2001). This project, which was funded by the Department of Health, included a survey of local authorities and voluntary organizations, supplemented with interviews with parents and carers in service user groups. The study found lots of activity and interesting work together with considerable commitment to the idea of user involvement. There were however a number of learning points which arose from the study. In particular there was confusion about what involvement means, only certain groups were consulted, and there was little idea about feedback to users or identifying what changed as a result of all the hard work. There was also little analysis of data and while most elements of effective involvement were in place, this was somewhat patchy in some local authorities.

While most of the above discussion centres on involvement at a more collective level in participating in planning decisions, user involvement also needs to be in place at the individual level – i.e. involving patients and carers in decisions about their own health and the care they give or receive.

Involving carers

User involvement needs to encompass carers as well as patients and service users. As the Department of Health (1999c) says, 'people who use services are in the best position to say how those services should be provided in order to meet their needs. Involving carers and their organisations, alongside patients and users of services, is a way to ensure that those services are responsive'. There are two aspects to this. Carers should be involved in planning and agreeing the care plan for the people they are caring for (subject to agreement with the person being cared for) and also in the planning and development of services: 'Too often', says John Bacon, London Regional Director of Health and Social Care, 'carers report that health and social care services do not include them or acknowledge their experience' (Carers Advisory Group 2001).

To involve carers effectively, organizations should develop a strategy for patient/user/carer involvement which has been agreed between local agencies, carers and service users. As the Carers Advisory Group (2001) says, this should include deciding how to involve carers and what help is available to encourage them to be involved. The latter might include help in arranging alternative care for the person they care for and payment for travel and alternative care costs. Specific action is also needed to encourage carers from ethnic minority communities to attend. Organizations should ensure that carers are represented on relevant committees, such as the local implementation teams for the Mental Health National Service Framework, and that the times and location of meetings suit carers. In addition they should provide training for staff on effective user and carer involvement, and monitor and review carer involvement.

The three Cs of user involvement

John Such, of Suffolk County Council Social Services Department, has identified three Cs of user involvement which are, he believes, essential to improve service quality through user involvement:

- *Commitment.* There needs to be real commitment to user involvement from councillors, senior managers, unit managers and staff. The easiest one to get, he says, is that of staff, as their priority is to improve services. However, managers frequently do not want to hear what they term 'negative views'. It is always easy to dismiss a particular group of users as unrepresentative. People may also point out, with justification, that the views of non-users are also important. However, John Such says 'let's get it right for users first, then attract more later'.
- *Cash.* This follows on from commitment. A budget to pay expenses to cover transport, costs of child care etc. is needed and there also needs to be an investment in advocacy services for people who can't speak for themselves, and in supporting user groups or groups of carers. Also, if funding is provided to a voluntary organization, they could be encouraged to involve their users or provide advocacy services. Training is another demonstration of commitment.
- *Communication.* User groups and user representatives should be treated with respect. Staff and managers must recognize that empathy and a plethora of relevant training courses are not sufficient. Staff cannot feel what they have not experienced. Users are the experts as they have experienced what it is like to be in their position. Meetings should be held at convenient times and the needs of the people taken into account. For example, to find out the views of people caring for children with disabilities it is not sufficient to ask if they can attend an evening meeting. Instead they could be invited, with the children, to a special lunch with people on hand to help with the children. Staff and managers could then talk to the carers (and indeed the children) in a relaxed setting, to get their views on the service and how it could be improved.

Responding to user views

Finally, responding to user involvement is not easy for managers and clinical professionals. Some groups may be very happy with the way the service is structured, but some may be opposed to the whole way the service is provided. Several mental health and maternity user groups fall into this category. In the former there is still an ongoing debate about the use of electroconvulsive therapy (ECT) and other interventions. In maternity services, pressure groups like the Association for the Improvement in Maternity Services are fundamentally opposed to the 'medical model' of birth for mothers who are well. Birth is not an illness, they argue, citing research indicating that it is safer for women who are well to give birth where they feel confident and relaxed. Managers and clinicians need to listen very carefully to these groups who may be very knowledgeable in their relevant field. As mentioned earlier, such groups could be dismissed as unrepresentative, but the only way to check is to go out proactively and listen to more users to get a fuller picture.

Beresford (2000) says that service users must be accorded the same respect as other participants in any discussions, 'without any imposition of stigma or assumption of their incapacity or inferiority, challenging rather than reinforcing dominant discriminations'. Moreover, recognition must be given to the subjective knowledge, analyses and perspectives of service users.

One organization invited some young people onto their selection panel for a key appointment. The managers on the panel, who were in a majority, all thought that a particular person was very suitable, but the young people did not like the candidate. After some heart-searching, the panel chair decided not to appoint, as she believed that was the commitment they made when inviting users onto the panel.

CHAPTER eight

Process improvement

It is no accident that the 'processes' box sits at the centre of the Excellence Model. An organization's processes are central to the experience of service users, patients and carers. It is through these processes that the other enablers are transformed into results.

Everything an organization does can be considered as a process. There is no product or service without a process. Harrington (1991) defines a process as follows: 'Any activity or group of activities that takes an input, adds value to it, and provides an output to an internal or external customer. Processes use an organisation's resources to provide definitive results'.

It is interesting that this definition uses the phrase 'adds value'. That is certainly the intention of a process. In practice, however, many processes may not actually add value. Sometimes a process can deliver negative value – for example, an over-complicated process for staff to apply for a place on a training course may actually deter staff from applying. One of the purposes of analysing processes is to make sure that they do add value; that each step of the process is important. If processes can be simplified, with no adverse effect on the customer, then that is an opportunity for improvement.

Processes can take many different forms. In health and social care they include surgery carried out on a patient, the process for approving someone as a foster carer, developing care plans, responding to requests for information, handling complaints, recruiting and interviewing staff, delivering meals and the process for allocating an individual worker to a specific client.

Coulson-Thomas (1994) distinguishes between three types of process. *Business processes* are sequences and combinations of activities that deliver value to customers. *Management processes* control and coordinate these activities and ensure business activities are delivered. *Support processes*, as the name implies, provide infrastructural and other assistance to business processes.

Redesigning the process

There are a number of steps in redesigning a health or social care process. As can be seen from the following list, process redesign is particularly relevant to the four Cs of Best Value: 'challenge' appears in Step 5, 'compare' in Step 3 and 'consult' in Step 4, while 'compete' is implicit in Step 5.

1 Define the process, its inputs and outputs, and draw a process diagram of the current process.
2 Look at existing measures of performance. What information do they give about the performance of the process?
3 Compare your measures of performance with those of other organizations, in health and social care or elsewhere, and see how they perform similar functions.
4 Consult with staff, patients, users, other organizations and people with an interest in the process.
5 With the aid of a facilitator, work with staff and other interested parties to identify ways of improving processes. Challenge the purpose of processes and individual activities and look for breakthrough improvements which can make a real difference.
6 Make sure that the organization is collecting the right performance indicators and other measures of the effectiveness of processes. Do they relate closely to the desired outputs?
7 Implement the changes.
8 Review progress against indicators, and go back to Step 1.

Defining the process

Step 1 above involves two main aspects: defining a process and drawing a process diagram. Defining a process involves identifying the desired outputs, the inputs and stakeholders. Figure 8.1 shows those for the process of a radiologist taking an X-ray of a patient. This process has a number of inputs, all of which are necessary for it to take place. There are two main outputs: the film for developing and, hopefully, a satisfied patient. In addition to the patient and the radiographer, relevant stakeholders may include doctors and other health professionals based at the hospital and at the GP surgery, the patient's family or carer, and possibly the X-ray maintenance department. In analysing the process it will be important to make sure that the views of all these people are taken into account.

As noted in the definitions above, a process will contain one or more activities. Some of these activities in the X-ray process involve the patient, some will involve the radiographer, while some will involve both. It is useful therefore to consider the process from the viewpoint of the different people involved and Figure 8.2 gives a simplified process diagram of the X-ray process, from the standpoint of the patient and from that of the radiographer.

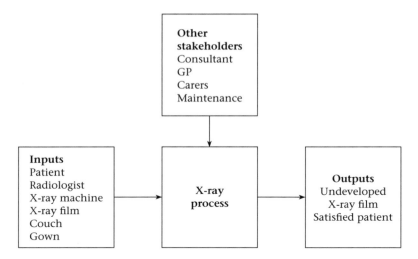

Figure 8.1 Defining an X-ray process

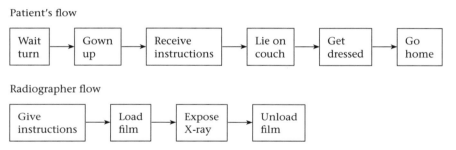

Figure 8.2 Process flow diagram for X-ray process
Source: Long (1996).

In addition it may be useful to draw a further flow series to illustrate the activities of the receptionist.

Certain activities (e.g. the radiographer giving instructions and the patient receiving them) by definition take place simultaneously, while the sequencing of many activities is fixed (e.g. the film cannot be exposed until it is loaded). However, there will also be some activities that could take place either sequentially or simultaneously. For example, the patient can be dressing at the same time as the film is being unloaded. Also the next patient can be gowning up at the same time as the current patient is being X-rayed.

This process flow diagram should be used to help investigate whether the desired outputs are achieved. In terms of the patient's sensual and psychological experience, it is important to analyse the interactions between the patient and the radiographer, in particular the information and reassurance given. The interactions between the radiographer and the machine are also important, in particular the operating procedures given and the ease of using the machine. Both of these aspects can improve the reliability of the process.

Writing down a process in this way can be a very helpful first step in analysing it with a view to further improvement. In some cases it can make people understand each other's roles in the process for the first time. Corinne Green, project manager of the Cancer Services Collaborative in Leicester, described the benefits of drawing up a map of the patient's journey as follows: 'We ran a brainstorming session with a range of people involved in the patient's "cancer journey": everyone from porters and clerks to clinicians . . . If you've worked with cancer patients for a long time, as I have, you think you know all the stages, but you don't. The visual map made us appreciate what an incredibly long and potentially difficult journey it is'.

Achieving breakthrough improvements

There are a number of ways a process can be redesigned to achieve breakthrough improvements. These include the following.

Making sure all activities add value

The definition of quality recommended in Chapter 1 refers to 'meeting the requirements and expectations of service users and other stakeholders *while keeping costs to a minimum*'. Making sure that all activities in a process add value, either directly or indirectly, to service users is often the key to keeping costs down without affecting the level of service provided.

In many cases, processes appear mysterious. They may be the result of custom and practice – 'we've always done this' – and in some cases no individual member of staff will know the whole process. In such cases, when a process diagram is drawn up, it may become immediately obvious that several stages do not add value or that by making one or two changes some activities are clearly redundant. In most cases activities that do not add value are an irritant to patients and service users, as well as taking up valuable staff time.

Improving processes at an ear, nose and throat clinic

The ear, nose and throat (ENT) clinic at Leicester Royal Infirmary discovered that patients went through a ten-stage process, as illustrated in Figure 8.3.

GP → Clinic → Waiting list → Admission office → Pre-assessment → Portered to theatre → Theatre → Recovery ward → Discharge by doctor → GP

Figure 8.3 Original process for ENT patients at Leicester Royal Infirmary

GP ⟶ Clinic ⟶ Theatre ⟶ Recovery ward ⟶ GP

Figure 8.4 Revised process for ENT patients at Leicester Royal Infirmary

This process was clearly not designed around the needs of the patient. Indeed, in some situations it was even worse as admission plans had to be deferred due to lack of bed space. The result was a lack of overall ownership or accountability, some duplication of effort, difficulties in scheduling, conflicts between elective and emergency demands and poor communications. Although the clinic was often rather fraught, there were also periods of relatively little activity.

The clinic addressed these problems by introducing day surgery for all patients with routine needs, enhancing the role of the GP in making an initial diagnosis, giving patients an information pack and discharging patients automatically following recovery where appropriate. The resultant process is shown in Figure 8.4 and consisted of just five stages rather than the original ten. In redesigning the process, it was identified that the processes eliminated did not add value. This resulted in meeting patients' needs better, while reducing costs.

Designing customized processes for particular groups

Many processes in health and social care deal with a wide variety of service users. In such cases instead of expecting all users, whatever their need or condition, to go through the same process, it may be better to design customized versions of the process to meet the particular needs of specific user groups. The ENT clinic above, which separated patients with routine needs from other patients, is an example of this. Another example is at the supermarket checkout. Instead of having all checkouts wide enough for a customer in a wheelchair, many will have one or two special 'wide aisles' clearly labelled whereas the rest can be narrower and allow the supermarket to have more checkouts. Most supermarkets also have one or two aisles designated for people with ten items or less. Since these customers are less willing to wait, this enables the supermarket to meet the expectations of different groups of customers more efficiently.

The radiology department, discussed earlier, may produce X-rays for emergency patients, inpatients and outpatients, with staff managing the workload by prioritizing staff according to clinical need. In such cases the waiting time for outpatients is likely to be excessive and it might appear impossible to improve this significantly without affecting the service for emergency patients. However, if instead there were separate processes for the three patient groups it would be possible to improve performance for each group. Figure 8.5 compares the two different situations – in the first all patients go through the same process while in the second there are tailored processes meeting the specific needs of each group.

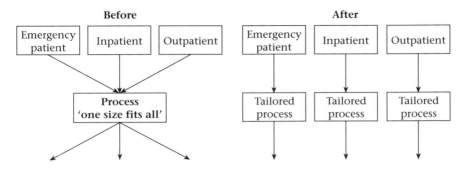

Figure 8.5 Customizing processes
Source: Based on Bevan (1997).

Another advantage of having separate processes for different patient groups is that it can allow for more flexible staffing. For example, one hospital's accident and emergency clinic opened a nurse-led minor injuries unit. This meant that highly trained (and expensive) doctors no longer had to deal with minor injuries that could be handled by specially trained nurses.

In social care, decisions about having separate processes for different client groups have been debated for many years. Should social workers in a locality team be generic – each social worker looking after some older people, some with mental health needs, along with some child protection work – or should they each deal with just one of these groups? The latter will allow them to specialize in a given field, while the former may give more flexibility if demands in the different groups vary through time. Also, there is the current debate on whether there should be specialist adoption and long-term fostering teams, or whether each social worker should do a mix of jobs in a 'permanence team'. While the former may allow greater focus and specialization, there is a problem concerning the perceived relative status and demands of the two roles.

Scheduling activities

Many tasks in health and social care are done in a step-by-step sequence – i.e. the second task is not started until the first one is completed. This is particularly common where different departments are involved. One example is in hospital discharge. A typical process in many hospitals is illustrated in Figure 8.6. Many hospital managers and doctors blame the social services department for patients occupying beds unnecessarily because discharge arrangements have not been finalized. However, if instead they had notified social services soon after the patient was admitted rather than waiting until the patient is medically fit for discharge, valuable bed space would be saved and the patient would be able to go home sooner. Another common reason for delayed discharge is that drugs that the patient needs to take out when

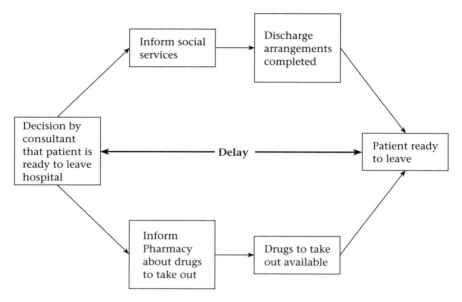

Figure 8.6 Typical process for hospital discharge

they leave are not available. Informing pharmacies in advance of patients' likely needs may reduce unnecessary delays.

Contemporaneous planning for children to be looked after is another relevant example. Rather than wait for the outcome of a high court hearing before beginning to look for a permanent home for a child, the search is initiated prior to the agreement from the court to the plan. Time is especially valuable in a young person's life.

A further example is the appointment of a new social worker, where often delays in receiving results from police checks may hold up the whole process. The personnel department may only request a police check when they have heard in writing that the candidate has accepted the post offered. If instead police were contacted as soon as the decision of the interview panel is known, the process could be speeded up. Another alternative is of course to get the police to improve their checking process which can take weeks or even months for a check which cannot take more than a few minutes of someone's time!

Identifying bottlenecks and constraints

No one will need reminding that there are a large number of constraints on decisions in health and social care, lack of resources being a fairly common one! However, in trying to improve performance it is important to analyse these constraints in detail to see if we cannot get round them in some way. For example, if we are trying to reduce trolley waits in a hospital or the time it takes to find a permanent solution for a child in foster care, we need to identify what factors and resources are the limiting ones. Only then can we begin to identify a solution. More detail on this topic is given in the next section.

Communication

In analysing processes, it is important to remember that many problems occur *between* processes rather than within a process itself. For example, the process for carrying out blood tests at a GP's surgery and that for analysing them at a nearby hospital may both be very good. However, if the process of delivering the blood sample to the hospital causes unnecessary delays, the overall service to the patient will be poor. It is important not to look at processes in isolation.

As well as analysing processes within a given department, it is important to identify, with staff from other departments or agencies, what happens to patients and users from their point of view. Many older people, for example, receive services from a variety of health and social care professionals. It will not be uncommon for an older person to receive services from the following in a given week: their GP, a district nurse, an occupational therapist, a home help and a physiotherapist at the hospital. While the individual processes may be well defined, without communication between the different professionals involved the older person is likely to get conflicting advice. Unless there is a coordinated plan for the person's overall care, the service will appear disjointed and each individual's best efforts will be undermined.

Goldratt's theory of constraints (TOC)

Goldratt's theory of constraints (TOC) described in the best seller *The Goal* (Goldratt and Cox 1993) addresses the challenges of dealing with bottlenecks and constraints in great detail. While Goldratt gives five stages, the theory of constraints is more easily considered in seven, as follows:

1 *Identify the goal or purpose of a system.* Without a clear goal, it is not possible to judge the impact of possible changes. Identify the main objectives and measures of performance.
2 *Identify the system's constraints and bottlenecks (the weakest link).* This involves prioritizing the constraints on the process. A system's constraints are anything that limits it from achieving higher performance in terms of its goals. For example, what are the limiting factors causing long waiting times for service users with a disability who are waiting for changes to make their home more accessible and convenient?

3 *Get the most out of the constraint.* Having identified the bottleneck, the next stage is to make sure it is worked as hard as possible since the throughput of the whole system will be limited by the throughput at the slowest step. For example, if time in operating theatres is at a premium it makes sense to consider how time in theatre is allocated to different clinics. In some hospitals where this is done in three-hour blocks, valuable theatre time can be lost when a particular clinic has fewer patients than normal and is not expected to use all its allotted time. Instead a more flexible allocation process would get more out of this constraint.

4 *Supporting the system's constraints.* This is about finding more creative ways of relieving the particular constraint. Decide how to exploit the system's constraints. Do not assume that constraints are here to stay. There is much we can do about them.

5 *Elevating the system's constraints.* Whatever the constraints are, there must be a way to reduce their limiting impact. There are many examples, particularly in health, where this concept has been used. For example, in managing ambulance services, if paramedics are in short supply it is not an efficient use of resources to have them taking patients for routine hospital appointments. Similarly if there is a shortage of social workers, identifying tasks that can be done by administrative staff, such as collection of statistics or writing up minutes, may relieve the bottleneck. Also, where resources are scarce, we need to ensure that they are used effectively. For example, if patients' notes are frequently not available at the start of a consultation with a doctor or therapist this will seriously reduce the throughput of the service.

6 *Remember that there are other initially less binding constraints.* Once we have tackled one constraint so that it no longer limits us as much as it did before, we may find that another constraint becomes more limiting. Further action to improve the original constraint will not improve the performance of the system unless the second constraint is also tackled.

7 *Once another constraint becomes limiting go back to Step 2.*

Figure 8.7 shows how the theory of constraints works. This is a simplified version of a patient flow series or pathway, and shows the maximum theoretical number of patients that can be processed at each stage. For example, the GP referral process could theoretically handle 100 patients per week,

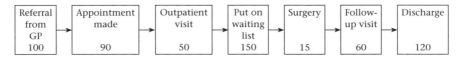

Referral from GP		Appointment made		Outpatient visit		Put on waiting list		Surgery		Follow-up visit		Discharge
100		90		50		150		15		60		120

Figure 8.7 Maximum capacities at each stage in a patient pathway
Source: Phipps (1999).

while a maximum of 60 follow-up visits could be made. In fact, only 15 patients per week can be handled because this is the capacity of the limiting constraint or bottleneck – in this case, surgery. Increasing the capacity of any other constraint will not speed up the process as long as the surgery stage remains incapable of increasing its throughput. Indeed, if more patients are admitted at earlier stages, all that will happen is that waiting times for surgery will increase.

Not recognizing a limiting constraint can have potentially dire consequences:

> The NHS has been praised for efficiency in having occupancy rates of 97 per cent and operating theatres and ICUs full to capacity at all times. Such lack of elasticity or tolerance in the system is actually bad for the Service and not accounted for by the supposed rise in emergency admissions or 'winter pressures'. It is the cause of patients lying on trolleys for hours on end, then going to inappropriate wards and waiting for space in the emergency theatre. Undoubtedly it leads to increased clinical risk to patients, poor quality care and sometimes unnecessary death.
>
> (Lugon and Secker-Walker 2001: 3)

Another important concept of Goldratt's is that of 'evaporating clouds'. Do not, he says, take a constraint as given. He cites the example of an organization's production line making a variety of different products. The organization must decide the 'batch size' – how many of each product to make in one batch before starting to make the next product. Ideally it would like small batch sizes to keep stock levels and costs low. However, the problem with this strategy is the time it takes to alter the production line whenever a different product is to be made. This time is known as the 'set-up time'. Many managers take this set-up time as given and work out the optimum batch size to balance set-up costs and inventory costs. However, instead the emphasis should be on finding creative ways, usually with fairly minimal investment, to reduce the set-up times themselves.

One of the main lessons from this example is that whenever we face a situation where it seems that a compromise is inevitable, we should always look to see if we can define the problem in a different way so that a simple solution that does not involve compromise becomes apparent. Goldratt (1990) says that 'there is *always* a simple solution that does not involve compromise', but in this author's naive opinion he may be overstating things a little!

Goldratt reminds us not to allow inertia (i.e. resistance to change) to cause a system constraint. In many cases finding the solution is the easiest part – it is getting solutions implemented and owned by relevant staff that is the difficult phase. It is important to recognize, Goldratt (1990) states, that any improvement is a change and that many (perhaps most) people perceive change as a threat to security. The consequence of this is emotional resistance which cannot be overcome by logic alone. The way forward is to try to create ownership of the idea by the group who have to implement it; to try to excite them about the fact that they are making an improvement.

Doing nothing is not an indifferent act. It is a conscious decision to ignore the problem and not to take appropriate action.

One of the best ways to see the interactions between different parts of any process is to develop a visually interactive computer simulation model depicting the system or the part of the system of interest. This will enable people to see the whole picture and evaluate the effects on the crucial performance measures.

Lean thinking

Another useful conceptual and practical framework for radically improving processes is that of lean thinking. Lean thinking is based on methods pioneered by Toyota and other Japanese companies to improve quality and reduce costs. Although originally applied to manufacturing, the ideas apply equally well to the service and public sectors.

A key aspect of lean thinking is identifying waste. Toyota identified seven different types of waste ('*muda*' in Japanese) (illustrated in Figure 8.8) (Hines and Taylor 2000):

- *Overproduction*. Producing too much or too soon, resulting in poor flow of information, people or products. An example would be producing large quantities of a drug which then becomes obsolescent.

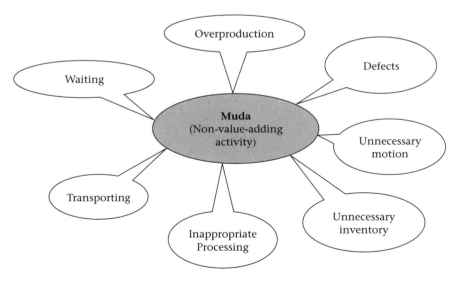

Figure 8.8 The seven types of waste

- *Defects.* Errors in paperwork or in the delivery of services and products.
- *Unnecessary motion.* Poor workplace organization resulting in poor ergonomics (e.g. excessive bending or stretching and frequently lost items).
- *Unnecessary inventory.* Excessive storage and delay of information or services, resulting in excessive cost.
- *Inappropriate processing.* Going about work processes using the wrong set of tools, staff, procedures or systems, often when a simpler approach may be more effective.
- *Transporting.* Excessive movement of people, information or goods resulting in wasted time, effort and cost. An example from a major UK shoe manufacturer is that leather travelled 22,000 miles during production – from Italy to the UK, to India and back to the UK. Examples in health and social care include patients moving unnecessarily from one ward to another and social workers visiting users who are not at home.
- *Waiting.* Long periods of inactivity for people, information or goods, resulting in poor flow and long lead times.

In their book *Lean Thinking*, Womack and Jones (1996) describe the essence of this approach in terms of five lean principles. These are given below, adapted slightly to emphasize their relevance to health and social care.

- Specify what does and does not create value from the perspective of service users and other key stakeholders, and not from the perspective of individual departments or organizations.
- Identify all the steps necessary to design and deliver services and products across the whole value stream to highlight areas which do not add value.
- Make those actions that create value flow without interruption or delays. This is particularly relevant where services are delivered by different departments or across different agencies (e.g. a laboratory that carries out blood tests quickly and efficiently, only for the results to take several days before being received by the commissioning clinic or GP).
- Only make what is 'pulled' by the customer. In manufacturing this means make to order rather than make to stock. In health and social care this translates to scheduling activities around the service user and not creating unnecessary delays.
- Strive for perfection by continually removing successive layers of waste as they are uncovered.

In a commercial environment it is easier to identify a value-adding activity – the key question is whether the customer would be happy to pay for it! In health and social care, such activities are those that, in the eyes of service users or other key stakeholders, make a product or service more valuable. It is recognized that some non-value-adding activities will be necessary and difficult to remove in the short term, but there will be many others that, with a little creative thinking and involvement of staff and service users, can be eliminated altogether.

As an example, patients with suspected prostate cancer at West Middlesex University Hospital saw a doctor in an outpatient clinic, returned on more than one occasion for a number of tests, and then again for their results. By redesigning the process to allow clinical assessment and the tests to be carried out during a single visit, with the results available the following week, the hospital was able to cut out many non-value-adding activities. As a result the time taken to identify a high risk of prostate cancer was reduced from six months to a maximum of 18 days.

Process improvement and business process re-engineering (BPR)

Business processes have been defined as sequences and combinations of activities that deliver value to customers (Coulson-Thomas 1994). There are two main approaches to redesigning those processes: process improvement and business process re-engineering (BPR). Process improvement tends to be more limited in scope and is generally easier to implement. Re-engineering is defined by two of the key proponents of BPR as 'the fundamental rethinking and redesign of business processes to achieve dramatic improvements in critical, contemporary measures of performance, such as cost, quality, service, and speed' (Hammer and Champy 1993).

The differences between process improvement and BPR are summarized in Table 8.1.

Some of the main benefits of BPR are that while service users are interested in the end-to-end or horizontal process, an organization can be focused

Table 8.1 Process improvement and BPR

	Process improvement	*BPR*
Scope	Part of a process within a particular function	Whole process, going across organizational boundaries
Mindset	As before	Fundamental rethinking, total redesign if necessary
Focus	Improving tasks	Eliminating delays between each step
Purpose	The need for the process goes unchallenged	Starts with the question: Should we be doing this at all?
Typical benefits	Improvements usually 5–20%	Targeted to deliver step change improvements of 50% in critical measures of process performance (e.g. cost, quality, speed)

inwardly and is managed through vertical lines of command. Also, as Talwar (1994) points out, 'To service the customer, work may have to flow across departmental divides. Each hand-off to another department introduces another potential source of delay in the process because the recipient department may be working to a different set of priorities'.

For example, patients referred by a GP for hospital treatment may experience excellent service from the GP who treats them with respect and makes an appropriate diagnosis. Similarly, when they get to the hospital, service may also be very good. However, while the GP surgery is well managed as is the hospital, there may be no one managing the interface between the GP and the hospital and the patient may experience poor service (e.g. long waiting times or poor communication between the two). Similarly, within the hospital the car park, reception staff and the different clinical disciplines are managed separately and there may be no one managing the experience of patients and carers when going from one area to another.

As Table 8.1 indicates, the main focus of BPR is eliminating delays. At one hospital, before using BPR, it took between seven and eight weeks for a patient to receive an appointment letter for surgery following the initial consultation with the consultant, and up to two years on the waiting list before being admitted to hospital. Now, following BPR, if the initial consultation shows that surgery is needed, a date is agreed the same day and the patient admitted to hospital typically around five weeks later.

BPR also tries to address over-complicated processes whose sole purpose is to check up on people to make sure they are not defrauding the organization or making mistakes. A large number of processes include a variety of controls and inspections, which are only there because the managers who designed the process did not trust their staff. Instead of incurring these extra costs day in and day out, BPR would put the emphasis on additional training, devolving responsibilities to staff so that they are empowered to make certain decisions without waiting for approval from their manager, and creating a supportive environment which allows people to learn from their mistakes. Changes can also be made to a process to make it less likely or even impossible to make a mistake. The Japanese call this *poka yoke*. In a manufacturing assembly process, for example, there may be two ways of assembling a product, one right and one wrong. A simple design change could remove the possibility of error altogether.

Many BPR projects involve the use of computing and IT. Up to date information is often the key to improving a process and IT can play a key role in this. In the early 1990s, there was a period where many projects were led by the IT department and did not deliver the required benefits. Nowadays it is accepted that projects should be led by the managers and people involved in the process, with IT playing a supporting and enabling role.

To conclude this chapter, a number of key principles of BPR, which have worked well in some other organizations, are given below (based on Coulson-Thomas 1994):

- Focus on service users and the generation of greater value for them. Many organizations appear to put more emphasis on internal customers than the beneficiary of the service.
- Give users a single and accessible point of contact through which they can harness whatever resources and people that are relevant to their needs and interests. The 'one-stop shop' that many public sector organizations have introduced in recent years is an example of this.
- Encourage learning and development by building creative working environments. Too many departments, in both private and public sectors, seem to put the emphasis on squeezing more out of people and working them harder, rather than improving the quality of working life and 'working smarter, not harder'.
- Concentrate on outputs rather than inputs, and link performance measures and rewards to customer-related outputs.
- Give priority to the delivery of value rather than management control. Empowerment is a key aspect of this.
- If the organization is structured on departmental lines, make sure that people meet other professionals and staff delivering service to the same group of users.
- Move discretion and authority closer to the service user.
- Encourage involvement and participation of both staff and users. Ensure people are equipped, motivated and empowered to do what is expected of them.
- Ensure that continuous improvement is built into implemented solutions.

PART three

Performance measurement

CHAPTER nine

Measuring performance

Measuring performance is a vital part of delivering excellence in health and social care. To deliver excellence, organizations need objective ways to measure how well they are doing and to monitor changes over time. Only then can they be sure whether previous changes have had a positive effect and find out which aspects of performance still need to be improved.

Organizations have of course always measured performance. Businesses have always looked at turnover and 'the bottom line'. Former nationalized industries such as coal and steel looked at output and costs. Other public services too have always had their own measures, often determined by central government or local councils. However, it is increasingly recognized that most measures organizations collect do not relate closely to the experience of their customers and clients. The number of patients treated or the number of cases processed, for example, are vital pieces of information but by themselves they tell us nothing about the quality of the services provided.

Measurement of performance must be clearly linked to the organization's strategy. If the organization is trying to deliver on its promises and really put patients and service users first, then it is vital that it measures what is important to each of these groups. It is also important that the measures chosen are seen as reasonable by staff. As the Department of Health's consultation document on *NHS Performance Indicators* (Department of Health 2001a) says: 'The choice of performance measures can have a major impact on the behaviour of people; credible performance measures can motivate them to improve, whereas poor measures may reinforce resistance to change'. For example, if a surgeon's performance is measured by comparing morbidity and mortality rates with other clinicians, then it will be difficult persuading surgeons to tackle high risk cases as then their performance rating is likely to fall. Instead, risk-adjusted methods are needed (Copeland 2001).

An illuminating example of the failure of performance measures to produce the required results is that of factories in the former Soviet Union which made nails. At first they were held accountable for the tonnage of nails produced. This led, not surprisingly, to a shortage of small nails and a surplus of large ones as it meant that fewer nails needed to be produced. Later the control was changed to the number of nails produced. Then, since it is cheaper to make smaller nails, there was a surplus of small nails and a shortage of large ones.

What is performance measurement?

The most quoted definition of performance measurement is that by Neely (1998): 'the process of quantifying the efficiency and effectiveness of past actions through acquisition, collation, sorting, analysis, interpretation and dissemination of appropriate data'. This definition makes explicit the need for a supporting infrastructure to acquire and analyse individual measures, together with a framework for assessing the performance of an organization as a whole.

However, a simpler definition, based on that of organizational excellence in Chapter 4, is given below. It shows clearly the relationship between achieving excellence and performance measurement. Without performance measurement it is impossible to assess the extent to which an organization delivers value and achieves excellence:

Excellence is outstanding practice in managing organizations and delivering value for customers and other stakeholders.

Performance measurement is evaluating how well organizations are managed and the value they deliver for customers and other stakeholders.

In designing a performance measurement system, a number of aspects need to be determined:

- what measures to use;
- why the organization needs to measure a particular aspect;
- how often it should be monitored (hourly, weekly, quarterly?);
- the level of detail required;
- who will collect the information and how;
- how reliable will it be;
- whether it can be fed directly into a computer for analysis;
- who should receive the information;
- how the information will be used.

While measurement is vital for effective management it is not an end in itself. If a particular measurement is invasive or reduces the quality of a customer's experience then it will need careful justification. Questionnaire overload is a factor here. Is the information really important? How accurate will the results be?

There is a danger at present that public services may be swamped with performance measures and it is important to evaluate the cost of collecting the information provided and to ensure that the benefits of additional indicators outweigh the costs of measurement. There is increasing evidence that the cost of measurement can be considerable. According to the Performance Measurement Association, Greater Manchester Police reported on Radio 5 that it costs them £22 million per year to collect the 92 best value indicators!

Sometimes the simplest measures are the best. For example, in a study on postnatal depression in the 1980s, clinicians asked patients a large number of questions about their lifestyle and feelings to see which indicators corresponded best with the clinicians' perception of whether a patient was depressed. The conclusion was that the simple question 'Do you feel you are depressed?' was a better indicator than any combination of the other indicators!

Aims of performance measurement

Performance measures are typically used in three ways:

- to review historic performance, answering the questions how well did we do and what do we need to improve;
- to encourage an improvement in performance, when used in conjunction with a reward structure;
- to directly bring about change, because someone who is monitoring performance within their control is likely to become intrinsically motivated to improve performance.

It is important to be clear about which of these uses is intended. They are not of course mutually exclusive and indeed a particular measure could be used with all three objectives in mind. Most self-assessment using the Excellence Model is ostensibly concerned with the first aim, although in practice the third aim is also present. Many of the performance measures introduced by government are associated with a reward system (or penalty system depending on which way it is looked at!). Best Value and the 'traffic light' system in the NHS Plan are examples of this, where authorities or trusts are rewarded or otherwise depending on the extent to which they meet the relevant criteria.

The third aim is a very common one and often essential in bringing about change. Indeed, Alan Underwood, former Deputy Chairman of the Royal Berkshire Ambulance Service, claims that 'Measuring performance is one of the strongest drivers for change'. For example, if a social work team is currently managed by making sure that individuals have a similar caseload (i.e. number of cases on their books), there is little incentive for them to process these cases more quickly as they will then be allocated extra cases to deal with.

Moreover, team spirit is likely to be poor, because some individuals will believe others are 'playing the system'. Trying to increase the speed of processing in such a team is doomed to failure unless the performance measures are related more to output and quality measures, rather than input measures. Moreover, if there was a common measurable goal which they could see related clearly to the experience of service users, team spirit would improve.

Neely (1998) describes the purposes of measurement in terms of 'four CPs':

- *CP1: check position.* This involves measuring to establish how well the organization is doing. Some people talk of 'corporate dashboards' telling managers where they are and the direction the organization is taking. Another aspect of this is to benchmark against other units or organizations and to monitor progress. Per Gunnar Andersson likens an organization with poor performance measures to a 'football team that keeps playing and playing but no one ever knows if it is winning or losing. No one would be motivated to play football'.

- *CP2: communicate position.* Government, the public and other stakeholders constantly want to know how well public sector organizations are doing. This is another purpose of performance measurement. Ideally the measures used should be the same as those used by the organization to check position, but in practice this is not always the case.

- *CP3: confirm priorities.* Performance measures can also identify differences between actual performance and targets. Once these differences are identified, the organization can develop action plans to close the gaps. As Neely (1998) says, 'without the measurement data there is no guarantee that appropriate action plans will be developed and no means of checking whether the proposed actions have their desired effect'.

- *CP4: compel progress.* Exhorting staff to improve performance on a particular aspect, without making any attempt to measure it, is often counterproductive and provides little incentive for staff to change behaviour. Measuring something gives a message that this aspect is important and is part of the process of improving performance. The measures used communicate priorities to staff and can motivate them to improve performance. The Department of Health (1998a) states that 'Any system for monitoring and assessing the performance of a service itself sends powerful messages about what the service is expected to deliver. For too long the emphasis has been on measuring activity, but this ignores some of the real needs of patients'. However, measurement by itself is not sufficient. Management need to discuss with staff how to improve performance on a given aspect and to act on the conclusions.

Benchmarking

While benchmarking is perhaps most closely related to Neely's CP1 (check position) it can also be useful in confirming priorities and compelling progress.

Benchmarking is a structured process of learning from the practice of others. It can be defined as continuously measuring and comparing one's processes against comparable processes in leading organizations to obtain information that will help the organization identify and implement improvements. The essence of benchmarking, as described in *The NHS Performance Assessment Framework* (NHS Executive 1999b) is 'the identification, understanding, dissemination and implementation of best practice'.

Benchmarking can take place at a number of levels:

- *Internal*: comparisons between different departments or areas within an organization (e.g. benchmarking older people and children's services in a local authority).
- *Competitive*: comparison of performance with similar organizations or departments (e.g. comparing the performance of occupational therapists at two different hospitals).
- *Functional*: comparison of one's own performance with other organizations performing similar functions within health and social care (e.g. benchmarking admissions procedures for cancer patients at one hospital with a different clinic elsewhere which is acknowledged to have developed 'best practice' admission procedures).
- *Generic*: comparison of one's own performance with others performing similar functions outside health and social care (e.g. NHS Direct benchmarking against a major call centre).

Benchmarking at the functional and generic levels can offer additional opportunities for improvement compared with competitive benchmarking. For example, a local authority wishing to improve its recruitment and retention of foster carers might learn much by comparing itself with another local authority. However, they might be more likely to identify radically different ways of operating by benchmarking against the processes used by the National Blood Service in its recruitment and retention of blood donors.

Why benchmark?

Oakland (1999) says that the main purposes of benchmarking are to:

- change the perspectives of executives and managers;
- compare business practices with those of world-class organizations;
- challenge current practices and processes;
- create improved goals and practices.

It is no coincidence that Oakland's list includes the first two of the four Cs of Best Value – challenge and compare (see Chapter 2). Benchmarking is an important part of Best Value. It opens up opportunities for creative thinking, rather than being internally focused and influenced by the fact that 'we have always done it this way'. Rather than just making incremental improvements, it helps the organization make real step changes and allows the possibility of transforming a poor performing area into one of the best:

> I have seen the benefits of benchmarking – within six months we made 120 improvements throughout 18 trusts. And I have always used benchmarking as a tool to ensure best evidence-based practice. It enables practitioners to sit down together in a supportive way to discuss what is best practice and what change process is necessary for them to deliver it.
> Paula Greenidge, deputy director of nursing and midwifery at
> Nottingham City Hospital

Carrying out a benchmarking study

There are a number of phases in a well-planned benchmarking study:

1 Identify the critical success factors for the department or organization.
2 Select processes for benchmarking. The processes chosen should have a significant impact on service users and the critical success factors.
3 Form a benchmarking team. This should include a 'process owner', a facilitator, people involved in the process and, if possible, user representatives.
4 Document the current process (use a flow chart) and develop meaningful performance measures.
5 Search for benchmarking partners. These could be within the organization, within health and social care or outside. Begin by agreeing on the criteria that partners should satisfy. Remember that benchmarking has value for both parties. Organizations approached are often very willing to participate.
6 Observe the partner organization(s), understand their processes, and collect relevant data.
7 Compare the organization and the partner(s). Identify gaps between the performance of one's own process and that of the benchmarking partner(s), and determine the root causes for any performance gaps.
8 Discuss these findings within the team and adapt the processes, taking into account information from the benchmarking study. Benchmarking is not about copying practices elsewhere, it is about learning, finding out how benchmarking partners do things and why.
9 Set new performance levels, objectives and standards that the new process should reach.
10 Implement the improved processes.
11 Monitor the results of the improvements.
12 Review the benchmarking process.
13 Maintain dialogue with the benchmarking partner and go back to Step 1.

Do not underestimate the importance of the preparatory work involved. As Andersen (1995) says, 'it might be tempting to rush the planning in order to reach the "real benchmarking", i.e. visiting partners, but the site visit is bound to be a failure if one turns up unprepared'. In particular, most value will be obtained if processes have been documented beforehand and meaningful measures developed to understand performance. Deming's theory of knowledge is very relevant here – an example of success cannot be successfully copied unless the underlying theory is understood (Deming 1993).

Choosing the right measures and ensuring that they are comparable is a vital part of the process. An NHS benchmarking club looking at absenteeism originally wished to benchmark against a Trust which had 4 per cent absenteeism, but later changed to one with 18 per cent absenteeism. The reason was that the two Trusts defined absenteeism differently: whereas the second Trust included lateness and long-term sickness in its definition of absenteeism, the other did not.

Other pointers for successful implementation of benchmarking include giving time to developing the relationship. Initially each party is likely to tell you their successes. A degree of trust is required before they will feel safe to tell it 'as it is'. It may also be useful to establish a process owner with the authority to go across functional boundaries to lead changes made as a result of the benchmarking study. It is also important to recognize that benchmarking is not a 'one-off' process but represents a commitment to a continuing process of performance improvement.

The performance prism

Performance measurement has been defined as measuring value to customers and other stakeholders. Of paramount importance therefore is measuring how well the organization meets the requirements and expectations of service users and other stakeholders. This will measure the outcomes for these stakeholders, however it is also useful to measure the effectiveness of the organization's processes and strategies, and whether it has the capability and capacity to deliver stakeholder requirements.

These factors are shown in the performance prism (see Figure 9.1), which shows the elements that a good performance measurement system should monitor. The prism also includes stakeholder contribution and involvement. This is particularly important for health and social care, where involving service users in decisions affecting their own care and in designing services to meet their needs is recognized as important in its own right, as is the involvement of partner agencies. It follows therefore that these aspects too should be monitored.

The main focus of the prism is the satisfaction of stakeholder requirements. In addition to measuring how well it is doing in meeting stakeholder requirements and expectations, the organization needs to evaluate whether it has appropriate strategies in place to meet these requirements and the ability of its processes to deliver. It also needs to identify whether it has the

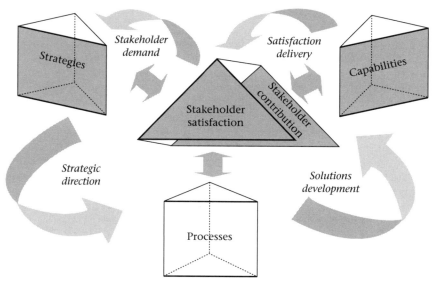

Figure 9.1 The performance prism
Source: Kennerley and Neely (2000).

capabilities (people, practices, technology and infrastructure) required to support and enhance these processes and whether they are being sufficiently nurtured and protected. Finally, the prism also recognizes that the contribution and involvement of stakeholders is a desired outcome and that this too should be measured.

Use of the prism at London Youth

The performance prism was implemented at London Youth, a charity whose aim is to provide, support and improve the range and quality of informal educational and social activities available to young people in the Greater London area. Its membership includes 460 youth clubs, groups and projects made up of 75,000 young people plus 5000 adult leaders and committee members.

The use of the prism can be illustrated using the 'success map' (Neely and Bourne 2000) built up during the development of performance measures in a series of workshops – see Figure 9.2. This shows the main stakeholders – young people, youth workers, youth club management committees, London Youth staff, funding bodies and regulators – and the main needs of each group. The success map also shows London Youth's main strategic aims (or intents) and their internal main business processes and capabilities.

After a number of workshops developing relevant performance measures for each aspect, an important further workshop took place which centred on

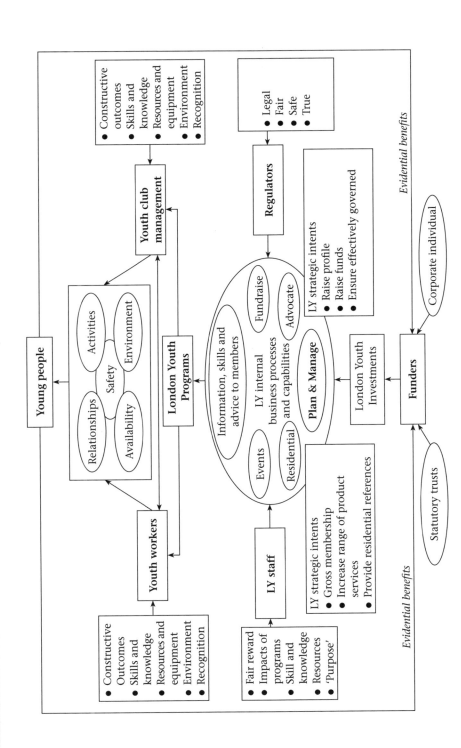

Figure 9.2 Success map for London Youth
Source: Neely *et al.* (2001: 7).

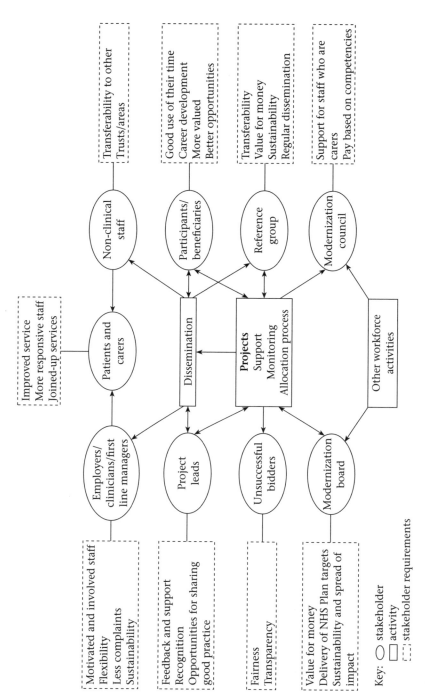

Figure 9.3 Success map for Trent Regional Health Authority's workforce taskforce

Key: ○ stakeholder
☐ activity
⌐¬ stakeholder requirements

Transferability to other
Trusts/areas

Improved service
More responsive staff
Joined-up services

Good use of their time
Career development
More valued
Better opportunities

Transferability
Value for money
Sustainability
Regular dissemination

Support for staff who are
carers
Pay based on competencies

Motivated and involved staff
Flexibility
Less complaints
Sustainability

Feedback and support
Recognition
Opportunities for sharing
good practice

Fairness
Transparency

Value for money
Delivery of NHS Plan targets
Sustainability and spread of
impact

Non-clinical
staff

Participants/
beneficiaries

Reference
group

Modernization
council

Patients and
carers

Dissemination

Projects
Support
Monitoring
Allocation process

Employers/
clinicians/first
line managers

Project
leads

Unsuccessful
bidders

Modernization
board

Other workforce
activities

'refining the measures selection and the process of converging on the "vital few" measures that the organisation felt were critically important and would be practically implementable, especially given its staffing and information technology constraints' (Neely *et al*. 2001). This is an important final stage to make sure that a performance measurement system is cost effective. Neely *et al*. also used a 'measures tree' to identify the essential linkages between the measures selected and each facet of the performance prism. In this way they could ensure that all facets were measured.

Measuring the effectiveness of a taskforce

The performance prism is also useful in measuring the effectiveness of quality improvement programmes. Figure 9.3 shows how it has been used to evaluate the work of Trent Regional Health Authority's workforce taskforce in commissioning projects for developing non-clinical staff (Moullin 2002). The first stage was to identify the key processes involved. These included allocating funds to projects, the support given and the monitoring process. A major aim was the sharing of best practice and another vital process was facilitating dissemination of the outcomes of the projects to other staff within the region. This process also needed to be evaluated.

In addition to looking at processes, it was essential to identify the relevant stakeholders and their main requirements. These included unsuccessful bidders, the project leads, a reference group set up to advise the taskforce, participants in the projects, other employers and staff who might learn from the projects, the modernization board which provided funds for the projects, and last but not least the patients and carers who will benefit from more effective non-clinical staff. A key stage in the evaluation was to find out directly from these stakeholders their main requirements and expectations of the taskforce, and then, on completion of the project, the extent to which these requirements were met.

One of the aims of the taskforce, as in most health and social care projects, was to make sure that key stakeholders participated and contributed to the project. Where there is an arrow in Figure 9.3 from a stakeholder to an activity, the evaluation considered to what extent the relevant stakeholder contributed to that activity. Finally, the evaluation needed to consider the extent to which the taskforce met its aims and whether in retrospect the taskforce adopted the right strategies and had the right capabilities to achieve these aims.

The balanced scorecard

Kaplan and Norton (1992) were concerned that traditional financial measures are only a guide to past performance and are insufficient for an organization that wishes to have a comprehensive picture of their business. CIMA (1993) agreed, saying that 'A focus on short-term traditional accounting measures such as profits, cash flows and inventory levels may no longer provide adequate indicators of good manufacturing performance'. Kaplan and Norton (1992) introduced the concept of the balanced scorecard, which they describe as follows:

> The balanced scorecard includes financial measures that tell the results of actions already taken. Also it complements the financial measures with operational measures on customer satisfaction, internal processes, and the organisation's innovation and improvement activities – operational measures that are the drivers of future financial performance.

The balanced scorecard has four different perspectives on the performance of an organization, all linked to each other (Kaplan and Norton 1996). These are:

- *The financial perspective*: how do we look to shareholders or other funding bodies?
- *The customer perspective*: how do we look to our customers?
- *The internal business perspective*: how good are our processes; what must we excel at?
- *The innovation, learning and growth perspective*: are we continuing to improve, learning from others and creating value?

Note that there are no specific measures given that an organization needs to include. Rather, it is for the organization to determine its main goals under each of the four headings and then to identify what measures of performance are most relevant to each of the goals. The scorecard should be linked closely to the strategic direction of the organization. Indeed, Kaplan and Norton (1996) claim that it should be possible to deduce an organization's strategy by reviewing the measures on its scorecard. The scorecard is used to drive change within the organization and is oriented towards the future, not the past.

The experience of Marks & Spencer (M&S) in recent years offers a salutary tale. Profits grew during the 1990s and in May 1998 the group had record profits. Surely a bright future was in store (pun intended!). However, if they had looked at other indicators, there were definite signs that the company would shortly be in trouble. Customer satisfaction with service had fallen – specifically the percentage of customers rating M&S' service 'good or better' dropped from 71 per cent in 1995 to 62 per cent in 1998, while the percentage saying that M&S' value for money was good or better dropped from 69 to 57 per cent in the same time period. As is well known, shortly after these record profit levels, sales fell while profits and share prices plummeted. It is clear that the indicators of customer satisfaction and value for money proved far more reliable than past profits in predicting future profitability. A balanced scorecard approach would have enabled the company to see more clearly the threats and difficulties much earlier.

Although widely used, the balanced scorecard has its shortcomings. In particular it does not put sufficient emphasis on the satisfaction of a number of stakeholders including employees, government, other agencies or the wider community. In some senses the scorecard is simply a recognition by accountants that financial performance measures do not tell them all they need to know – a fact that has been recognized by many other professions, including quality management, for many years. Nevertheless, the basic principle of the scorecard – that performance needs to be measured using a balance of measures – cannot be disputed. Another key lesson from the balanced scorecard is that it is wise to keep the number of measures in each box fairly small. This will enable the organization to see clearly how it is doing on its major dimensions without being distracted by large numbers of subsidiary performance measures.

A balanced scorecard for public sector organizations

In health and social care, even more than in private industry, the need for a balanced set of measures is paramount. All the concerns of private companies apply, but with an additional set of public sector values – for example, equality and fairness. As Nicholls *et al.* (2001) say: 'Health care professionals need to design and use balanced sets of measures which cover clinical effectiveness, patient experience, risk management effectiveness, resource effectiveness and strategic effectiveness'.

The need for a balanced set of measures is an integral part of both Best Value and the NHS Performance Assessment Framework. Best Value has five measures (strategic objectives, cost/efficiency, service delivery outcome, quality and fair access), whereas the Framework has six (health improvement, fair

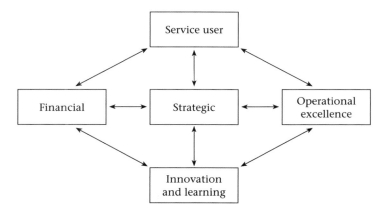

Figure 9.4 The five perspectives of the Public Sector Scorecard
Source: Moullin (2002).

access, effective delivery of appropriate health care, efficiency, patient/carer experience and health outcomes of NHS care).

While Kaplan and Norton's (1996) balanced scorecard can be applied to the public sector, the headings used do reflect its private sector origins. The Public Sector Scorecard illustrated in Figure 9.4 (Moullin 2002) was designed specifically for the public and voluntary sectors. This has five perspectives. The strategic perspective refers to the key performance outcomes reflecting why the service exists and what it seeks to achieve. The service user perspective is concerned with how the organization looks to service users and other key stakeholders. The operational excellence perspective refers to the effectiveness of processes and of staff and includes measures such as staff satisfaction. The financial perspective refers to how well the organization manages its funds and keeps costs down, while the innovation and learning perspective looks at whether it is continuing to improve, learning from others, and creating additional value for service users and other stakeholders.

An example of how the Public Sector Scorecard can be used is given in Table 9.1, although in practice there will be additional measures under each perspective. The table shows clearly the link between measurement and strategy – the final column being concerned with how the organization aims to achieve its targets.

Table 9.1 Example of a completed public sector scorecard

	Objective	*Measure*	*Target for the year 2002*	*Initiative: action required*
Strategic	Provide service to more users	No. of service users	2001 767 2002 830	Reduce delays
Financial	Reducing cost	Cost per user	2001 £75 2002 £70	Reduce unnecessary visits
Service user	High user satisfaction	Survey measure	2001 63% 2002 70%	Address customer service issues
Operational excellence	More staff training	% of staff on courses	2001 46% 2002 70%	Train staff on key issues
Innovation and learning	Improve user awareness of services	% of users aware of service (survey)	2001 not recorded 2002 75%	Roadshow in town centre

Measuring performance using the Excellence Model

The Excellence Model incorporates many of the attributes of the balanced scorecard. Like the scorecard, the Excellence Model has four results categories or measures: customer results, employee results, society results and key performance results. Innovation and learning, while not a results category, is a key element of the Excellence Model. In addition, the Excellence Model does not just measure the results categories, it also measures an organization's effectiveness on each of the enabler categories using RADAR (see Chapter 4).

When Salford Royal Hospitals Trust began to use the Excellence Model, they discovered how little information available was suitable for a clinical organization that wanted to put clinical quality at the heart of its management processes (Pavlou and Chisnell 1997). Most of the information systems were clearly designed to support the finance function rather than the clinical function. This highlighted the need to develop a new set of performance indicators, based on the Excellence Model. These included:

- clinical results chosen by the Trust's clinical staff as important and meaningful;
- ease of access to clinical services, such as waiting times;
- the financial base on which the clinical services are founded;
- levels of satisfaction of patients, referring clinicians, purchasers and staff;
- the contribution of the Trust to the local, national and international community.

Perception measures, performance indicators and outcomes

The Excellence Model differentiates between perception measures and performance indicators when assessing people results, customer results and society results. *Performance indicators* are internal measures collected by the organization in order to monitor, understand and improve its performance. *Perception measures* reflect the views of members of staff, customers or society. They come directly from these groups and can be obtained from customer surveys, focus groups, complaints and compliments.

Both are important. The example given in Chapter 3 of a rail company wishing to monitor delays makes this clear (see p. 67). It could measure the delay between trains arriving at their destination compared with the scheduled time. This is a performance indicator. It will be fairly easy to collect and the rail company will easily be able to show whether delays are being reduced or not. However, it will not be able to establish, using this indicator alone, how customer satisfaction with journey times has changed over the same period. For example, people on a long journey may be happy if a train is up to ten minutes late, but those commuting a relatively short distance may be very dissatisfied. If however the company also asked customers directly via a self-completion questionnaire how satisfied they were with journey times (a perception measure) it would get a much better perception of service quality.

People's expectations are also constantly changing. What people were satisfied with two years ago may now be seen as very poor service. For example,

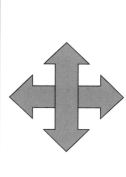

People results

Perception measures
Satisfaction with meaningfulness of work, variety, autonomy, communication, empowerment and role clarity. Feeling supported by managers and leaders. Satisfaction with pay, rewards and physical working conditions.

Performance indicators
% of employees on training courses, absenteeism, employee turnover, equal opportunities.

Society results

Perception measures
Views of local people on the unit's employment policies, involvement in the community and environmental policies. Stigma associated with admission to unit.

Performance indicators
Environmental and waste policies, evidence of support for employee initiatives in the community, raising social awareness of mental health issues.

Customer results

Perception measures
Satisfaction with admission and diagnosis, quality of accommodation including privacy, the day schedule and activities, quality of treatment and care – as measured by surveys and exit interviews. Also feedback from visitors and referrers.

Performance indicators
User complaints and compliments, performance against national standards.

Key performance results

Outcomes
Costs versus budget, staff cost per occupied bed, admission rates, discharge rates, waiting times for admission, number of readmissions, quality of care (e.g. measured by a quality of life index).

Indicators
Financial management, patients treated, duration of stay, process improvement.

Figure 9.5 Measuring performance in a mental health unit using the Excellence Model

a GP practice may find that the average waiting time for patients (a performance indicator) has reduced from 25 minutes to 20 minutes over a two-year period. However, whereas people may have been satisfied with waiting for 25 minutes in a GP surgery in the past, the surgery might find that even a 20-minute wait is now seen as unacceptable. If in addition to monitoring average waiting time, the surgery asked patients for their perceptions on whether they thought the delay was excessive it would get a much clearer picture. A survey by itself, however, would not give surgery staff information about what has been happening in the past and would not provide sufficient guidance about what needs to be done. Both perception measures and performance indicators are needed.

While perception measures and performance indicators are used for the first three results categories, key performance results are assessed on performance outcomes and indicators. Performance outcomes are the main results required by an organization and its key stakeholders.

Using the Excellence Model to measure performance in a mental health unit

Figure 9.5 illustrates how the Excellence Model can be used to measure the performance of a unit providing inpatient and outpatient services for elderly patients with mental health needs. This figure shows only the results categories. In addition, the unit would measure its effectiveness in relation to the enablers of the model: leadership, policy and strategy, people, partnerships and resources, and processes.

Quality performance indicators

As organizations move away from traditional approaches of management towards continuous quality improvement and other more customer-oriented approaches, the measures of performance they use need to reflect their changing priorities. Traditional measures of quality and performance have a number of weaknesses for measuring service quality. They are often inwardly focused rather than focused on patients and service users. They also emphasize output and machine or server utilization much more than quality. For example, focusing on the utilization of beds in a hospital, while useful, has several weaknesses. Beds may be occupied because discharge arrangements or drugs that are needed to take home are not available, or because a patient needs to see a consultant whose next visit is on Friday.

Another problem with conventional measures is that they tend to be focused on some cost centres but not others. Who, for example, measures the performance of the invoicing department or the personnel department? Instead, organizations need to measure the effectiveness of individual processes within the organization.

Table 9.2 Quality performance indicators at Federal Express

Type of error	Weight
Lost packages	10
Damaged packages	10
Wrong day late	5
Package status unavailable from tracking system	3
Complaints reopened	3
Right day late	1
Missed proof of delivery	1
Invoice adjustments	1
International operations	1

Quality performance indicators are a very useful way of measuring service quality, avoiding many of the above problems. As the Department of the Environment, Transport and the Regions (DETR) point out: 'Without a rigorous basis for collecting and presenting performance against key indicators, and a real sense of the ownership of the information that is published, there is a risk that resources can be diverted from the issues that matter most to those at the sharp end of service delivery' (DETR 1998). Whereas there could be a large number of indicators for an organization, it is recommended that there are no more than ten for a given team. A performance indicator can be defined as a valid and reliable quantitative process or outcome measure related to one or more dimensions of performance.

It is useful at this stage to look at the quality performance indicators used by Federal Express (see Table 9.2). Several points can be noted from these. First, the majority of the indicators relate to factors important to the customer: if a package is lost, late or damaged, if the company cannot locate it when the customer enquires, if complaints have not been dealt with to the satisfaction of the customer. Second, the indicators measure the performance of departments like customer services, invoicing and computer services which are not normally monitored. Finally, the indicators are given weights determined by feedback from customers to reflect their relative importance in customers' eyes.

Developing quality performance indicators

Most organizations develop measures in a fairly haphazard way, adding new ones when existing ones do not provide what is required. However, there are many advantages in developing quality performance indicators in a systematic way. In particular it ensures that all important areas are measured and avoids the temptation to ignore aspects that are important but difficult to measure.

The following five stages are recommended for developing quality performance indicators. If possible, involve both staff and service users at each stage:

1 Identify service users and others with an interest in the service and determine their requirements and expectations.
2 Define the work process that provides the service.
3 Define the value-adding activities and outputs of the process.
4 Develop performance measures related to each activity.
5 Evaluate the performance measures to determine their usefulness.

In order to evaluate performance indicators for an organization or department, it is important to ask the following questions: are they focused on service users and other stakeholders, do they reflect all the value-adding activities of the organization or just a few of them and do they measure the quality of all the various processes in the organization? Finally, do the benefits of additional indicators outweigh the costs of collection?

The following case study, based on the work of Alan Power of Lloyds TSB, shows how TSB Homeloans have used this framework to develop performance indicators for their business.

Performance Indicators for TSB Homeloans

Stage 1: Identify all customers and their requirements

Those with a stake in the mortgage system include:

- the borrower;
- the retail branch for whom the borrower was their customer;
- the central marketing department, who developed products, decided price (mortgage rate etc.) and carried out promotions;
- the central risk management department who determined lending policy or criteria;
- the borrower's solicitor;
- the bank's life and pensions company, who offered collateral security for the loan;
- the bank's general insurance company, who offered a series of related products (e.g. building and contents insurance, payment protection insurance).

Some examples of the service requirements of the stakeholders are:

- issue offer of mortgage within five days of receiving completed application documentation from the retail branch;
- reply to borrower's after-sales service enquiries within ten working days;
- reply to solicitor's request for redemption quotation within five working days.

Stage 2: Define the work process that delivers the service

TSB Homeloans then examined the processes needed to deliver the service levels required. Four areas were covered:

- customer actions which come into contact with the two types of employee action listed below;

Table 9.3 Quality performance indicators for applications processing

Error type	Weight
Application form incomplete	1
MIRAS form incomplete or missing	5
Valuation incomplete or missing	5
References or credit references not enclosed	3
Right-to-buy forms not enclosed	3
Uplift documents not enclosed	3
Checklist or control sheet not enclosed or incomplete	1
Life insurance/general insurance details missing	2
Manager's recommendation unclear	1
Writing unclear	1

- on-stage employee actions which are visible to the customer (e.g. staff in the retail branch);
- backstage employee actions that are not visible to the customer but directly affect customer satisfaction;
- support processes which are all other processes which support the frontline staff, including marketing, IT and credit management.

Stage 3: Defining the value-added activities and outputs of the process

The company then identified where value may be added to customers. Five key business drivers were defined as 'value-adding':

- applications processing;
- completion processing;
- after-sales service;
- redemption processing;
- further advance processing.

For each process the output was defined in terms of the deliverables and the service standard.

Stage 4: Developing performance measures

Performance measures were applied to each of the key processes. Those for applications processing are shown in Table 9.3. The weighting indicated the significance of the error (e.g. a weight of 5 was applied to anything that was a 'fatal' error, whereby the processing of the application could not proceed without the error being rectified). The data was monitored monthly using control charts. Similar methods were used to measure the performance of the four other key business drivers.

Stage 5: Evaluate the performance measures

TSB Homeloans then evaluated the performance measures to determine their usefulness. They found that this approach was successful in identifying the type of errors and their frequency. This in turn offered opportunities to engage in improvement activities using such tools as cause and effect diagrams and brainstorming.

Best Value performance indicators

As mentioned in Chapter 2, performance measurement is one of the key areas of Best Value. Best Value classifies performance indicators into five dimensions:

- *Strategic objectives*: why the service exists and what it seeks to achieve.
- *Cost/efficiency*: the resources committed to a service and the efficiency with which they are turned into outputs.
- *Service delivery outcomes*: how well the service is being operated in order to achieve the strategic objectives.
- *Quality*: the quality of the services delivered, explicitly reflecting users' experience of services.
- *Fair access*: ease and quality of access to services.

Examples of performance indicators under each heading are shown in Table 9.4. Note that some indicators are in fact perception measures.

Measuring user perceptions

Measuring and monitoring customer satisfaction is a vital part of a quality management programme. How can an organization establish how well it is doing without taking systematic steps to measure customers' perceptions of the service? As Donabedian (1980) says, 'client satisfaction is of fundamental importance as a measure of the quality of care because it gives information on the provider's success at meeting those client values and expectations which are matters on which the client is the ultimate authority'.

In contrast, many service organizations, in health and social care and elsewhere, make little real attempt to monitor customer satisfaction. Others collect information on certain aspects of their service but either do not analyse it fully or do not have a process for translating this feedback into action. There are several reasons why organizations do not find out what customers want and expect and how they perceive the service provided. First, many managers and staff believe they already know what the customer wants. They may be right, but the only way to be sure is to ask the customers themselves. Second, some managers assume that if no one complains then the service must be OK. However, it is well known that in the UK few people who experience

Table 9.4 Examples of Best Value performance indicators

Strategic objectives	Percentage of children looked after with three or more placements during the year. Percentage of young people leaving care aged 16 or over with at least one GCSE (grades A*–G) or GNVQ. Percentage of children on the child protection register who had been visited at least once every six weeks by their social worker.
Cost/efficiency	Cost of services for children looked after. Cost of intensive social care for adults.
Service delivery outcomes	Number of households receiving intensive home care. Older people aged 65 and over helped to live at home. Number of funded day centre places for people aged 75 and over.
Quality	Clients receiving a review as a percentage of adult clients receiving a service. Percentage of items of equipment costing less than £1000 delivered within three weeks. User satisfaction with the home care service. Percentage of people receiving a statement of their needs and how they will be met.
Fair access	Percentage of people surveyed who said that they felt matters relating to race, culture or religion were taken into account by social services in the provision of the help they needed. Proportion of local authority owned passenger transport vehicles adapted for passengers with special needs.

a problem will complain. Indeed this has been given as one of the main reasons that UK service quality is poor. A third reason why organizations do not listen to customers is that they are not really interested. 'We've always done it this way', they say, and then when someone complains they say: 'No one else has complained', the implication being 'What's wrong with you?'

It is, however, relatively easy to find out how users and carers perceive services – just ask them! Whichever method is used to elicit user views, it is important to go through a number of steps to get the best return on the money, time and energy invested:

1 Review existing research and feedback. This is an important step, but one which is often ignored. Previous research may have found the information needed already and will at least help avoid the mistakes of previous attempts.
2 Determine the objectives, time scale and budget. Ensure that there is commitment from management to act on the results. Some managers design a questionnaire with the aim of getting a high rating from their users!

3 Decide what, where and when to measure. Which groups should be questioned? Make sure that measures examine what is important to service users. Avoid information overload and keep it simple.
4 Decide sample size and research methodology. Sample size is often a major determinant of cost, but small samples may not be reliable.
5 Conduct the research.
6 Analyse and interpret the results.
7 Disseminate the results and work closely with those involved in providing the service to develop a plan of action for service improvements.

There are a number of ways to open up service user access to organizations in health and social care. These include the following (adapted from Martin 1989):

- Get out and talk face to face with patients, carers and other service users. Get to know them.
- Organize focus groups. Invite selected users to come in and discuss what they like and dislike in an open forum.
- Ask users to respond to a survey.
- Have suggestion boxes and feedback forms available in strategic places (e.g. in surgeries, community centres, hospitals).
- Initiate a newsletter or other communication device to broadcast how much the service wants the input of users and how it will respond to it.
- Move customer service communication and complaint handling from a low priority in the organization to one with clout. The NHS Patient Advice and Liaison Services are an example of this.
- Respond, respond, respond – and rapidly – to all complaints, compliments and requests.
- Provide customers with help and encouragement in making complaints and compliments (e.g. a freephone number). Remember many users will feel intimidated and will worry that they will be treated badly if they complain. One idea, which might fit in well with the NHS modernization programme's theme 'making a difference' would be to invite patients and carers to say either what made a difference for them (i.e. their expectations were exceeded) or what *would* have made a difference.
- Measure and evaluate managers' performance on the ability to obtain feedback from users.

Two methods of gathering information from users – qualitative methods and questionnaires – are analysed in more detail below.

Qualitative methods

Qualitative methods include focus groups and user panels, both of which seek to find out users' feelings and attitudes on an in-depth basis. There are many examples of this within health and social care. Usually the format is that a group of users are invited to attend an informal meeting where they offer their opinions on the quality of the service provided, together with possible areas for improvement. It is important that expenses are paid in order to encourage people to take part. It is also important to take note of what people say and to report back to them what actions have been taken as a result. Otherwise participants will consider it a waste of their time.

BT is one of several commercial companies to use customer liaison panels to get customers' views (others are Safeway, Boots and the Nationwide Building Society). These panels are composed of three BT staff and between 9 and 12 people from the local community who have been identified as key local network individuals by an external market research agency. They have a two-hour meeting every two months to discuss subjects such as payphones, complaint handling, marketing policies and phone books. Members are not paid as such but do receive expenses together with Prestel equipment to stay in touch with each other between meetings and get access to BT information and the minutes of meetings in other districts.

Jan Walsh, Corporate Customer Relations Manager, receives reports of all panel meetings. She says that apart from financial advantages there are a number of other pay-offs to the company: 'The principles of cooperation and participation that the panels have developed extend into other management areas so that the company is focusing more on managing the customer's experience. You create an environment where customers and managers get together regularly to share the objectives and outcomes that both want. This all helps to move the company towards being customer-driven' (Hopson and Scally 1991).

The critical incident technique

Another qualitative method to gain information from users is the critical incident technique. This involves asking users simple open-ended questions, usually in face-to-face situations, about their particular experiences in a recent incident or interaction with the organization. The critical incident technique can be particularly useful in obtaining the views of children. Getting accurate perceptions from children is notoriously difficult, however there has been some pioneering work in this area by the National Society for the Prevention of Cruelty to Children (NSPCC).

The NSPCC wished to explore the views of children who had experienced the protection services they provide. Children and young people aged from 5 to 17 were asked to think about their experiences of the NSPCC and to describe any incidents which they found to be either helpful or unhelpful. The following examples (Dotchin 1994) illustrate the power of some of the statements obtained using this technique:

> The social worker gave me a piece of paper with a number on it in case I needed to get in touch with her. I hid the number away.

> I was not asked if I would like to be on my own – it's better on my own.

We got told off at school for being late. I wanted the NSPCC to explain to school we were up late waiting for dad. They didn't do this.

When I first visited the NSPCC I thought that the inside of the building looked like a nursery and I felt I did not fit in. I felt uncomfortable and would have preferred a room more like a lounge.

I hated notes being taken on the first interview and wondered who they were for and who was going to see them. Did the whole world know what was happening to me?

The NSPCC also encourage children to give feedback via a specially designed computer program to capture their views. This puts them in control and has increased response rates dramatically.

Questionnaires

More and more organizations are using questionnaires to evaluate their service – however, they are not always well designed. 'Anyone can design a good questionnaire' is a common misconception. It requires considerable skill and experience. The starting point is to be clear about what the organization requires from the questionnaire. One needs to ensure there are no ambiguities, no loaded questions, and that the questionnaire is no longer than necessary. The questionnaire should be pre-tested with a pilot survey to make sure it works well. One large teaching hospital produced what in many respects was a well-drafted questionnaire and asked whether patients were satisfied or not (using a five-point scale) with each of a number of aspects of the service provided. However, it was apparent that staff had thought up the questions themselves without first finding out what mattered most to patients. A face-to-face pilot survey on a small number of patients would undoubtedly have identified this.

One of the first decisions to make is how to administer the questionnaire. Should it be face to face, by telephone, by post or self-completion made available to the user on the organization's premises?

Face to face interviews

Face to face interviews are more expensive than other methods. However, they give quicker response and can be longer and less structured than other forms of questionnaire. Interviewing is an undervalued skill. Interviewers need to be trained in how to ask questions and interpret answers, without biasing the results.

As with other methods it is important to decide who to interview. South Yorkshire Police had two main choices in their annual survey. One option was to interview a sample of residents in South Yorkshire. However, this sample would contain many people who had no contact with the police in the last year or so and would therefore not provide them with up-to-date data. The second option, which they adopted, was to try to interview every-one who had had some interaction with South Yorkshire Police in a particular week. This was particularly useful since, like health and social care, people's perceptions of the police are heavily influenced by the media.

Telephone interviews

This is becoming increasingly common, with names drawn at random from the telephone directory. It is cheaper than face-to-face interviews, however the re-sponse rate may be lower and this method irritates some people. Attention needs to be given to the following when administering a telephone questionnaire:

- Telephone subscribers themselves form a biased sample. People who share a telephone and those on low incomes are under-represented. Also, some groups are more likely to be in when the caller rings. The timing of the call, day or evening, may bias the sample.
- What about situations when there is no answer? How many recalls should be made? This may also bias the sample.
- Who should the caller ask for? What if children or relatives answer?
- What if, as is common, the respondent objects to using the telephone in this way or simply refuses to answer?

Postal questionnaires

Postal surveys are easy to organize and can be fairly cheap if response rates are high. More usually, however, response rates for postal questionnaires are in the region of 15 to 20 per cent unless an incentive is given, compared with up to 85 per cent for face-to-face interviews. Also, there is a greater risk that the respondent does not fill in the questionnaire very accurately and it may take a period of time before most questionnaires are returned.

In designing a postal survey it is important to get an accurate list of names and addresses and also to keep the questionnaire relatively short and easy to complete. Attention should also be given to the accompanying letter.

Self-completion questionnaires

Self-completion questionnaires are probably the most common method for gaining feedback from customers. They are typically made available at the point where service is provided, but could be available elsewhere. The advant-ages of self-completion questionnaires is that they are cheap to administer and also give a message to customers that the organization is interested in listening to their views and, by implication, in improving the service pro-vided. One disadvantage is that they do not find out what non-users think about the service. Also, there is no guarantee that the questionnaires com-pleted are representative of all customers. Some pointers to the successful use of self-completion questionnaires are:

Birmingham
Midshires
Building Society

Gaining Customer Input
How satisfied are you that we are:

		Exceeded Expectations	Highly Satisfied	Satisfied	Dissatisfied	Highly Dissatisfied
Friendly	– *the process we use is businesslike and friendly*	O	O	O	O	O
Informed	– *we give you the information you need*	O	O	O	O	O
Responsive	– *available and dependable when you need us*	O	O	O	O	O
Service-orientated	– *easy to do business with*	O	O	O	O	O
Trustworthy	– *honest, responsive and ethical*	O	O	O	O	O

	Yes	No
Would you make us First Choice?	□	□
Would you recommend us as First Choice?	□	□

Figure 9.6 Measuring customer perceptions at Birmingham Midshires Building Society

- include a statement, perhaps from a senior manager, explaining the benefits of completion;
- pay attention to the layout of the questionnaire, making it easy to complete, and keep it short;
- ensure that return of the questionnaire is made easy: a freepost address or a posting box clearly marked on the organization's premises;
- remember to thank customers for their participation in the survey.

An example of a well-designed self-completion questionnaire is that developed by Birmingham Midshires Building Society, which was named 'The UK Service Excellence Company of the Year' by Unisys/*Management Today* in 1996. As can be seen from Figure 9.6, the link between their values – friendly, informed, responsive, service-oriented and trustworthy – and the performance measures is clearly shown. It also requests information on re-purchase intentions, although in health and social care a measure of overall satisfaction would be more appropriate.

The main advantages and disadvantages of the different methods of administering questionnaires are given in Table 9.5.

Table 9.5 Advantages and disadvantages of different questionnaires

Method	Advantages	Disadvantages
Face to face	Quicker response Can be better structured and longer	Expensive Interviewer bias
Telephone	Relatively cheap	People can get irritated Response rate typically lower Some groups will be under-represented
Postal	Easy to organize Fairly cheap	Typically low response rate Responses may be less accurate Can only ask relatively simple questions May take a long time to get responses back
Self-completion	Very cheap Gives the message that the organization wishes to listen	Only covers users, whereas the organization may also be interested in non-users or infrequent users

Analysing questionnaires

Many organizations with well-designed questionnaires get relatively little out of the survey due to poor analysis. For example, feedback on overall patient satisfaction at a GP surgery revealed that 7 per cent of patients reported they were very dissatisfied, 12 per cent dissatisfied, 68 per cent satisfied, and 13 per cent very satisfied. This data could be summarized in two different ways: 'Over 80 per cent of patients were satisfied or very satisfied with the service overall' or 'Nearly 20 per cent of patients were either dissatisfied or very dissatisfied'. Both statements are correct, but they give different messages – one of complacency and the other that there is much work to be done.

In analysing such a questionnaire it is important to establish the general aim. If the organization wishes to move towards excellence, the aim must be to get as many patients as possible in the very satisfied category. It follows that the greatest benefits will come from establishing what aspects of the service those who were not satisfied overall were unhappy with and addressing these. Also, finding out more about the experiences of those who were very satisfied can help identify what the organization is doing right and enable it to make sure that this happens more frequently.

Table 9.6 Measuring user perceptions and expectations

	Strongly agree						Strongly disagree
Expectations Patients/service users should have a wide range of choice regarding meals	1	2	3	4	5	6	7
Patients/service users should be involved in determining their care plan	1	2	3	4	5	6	7
Perceptions I had a wide variety of choice regarding meals	1	2	3	4	5	6	7
I was involved in determining my care plan	1	2	3	4	5	6	7

Measuring perceptions and expectations

As mentioned in Chapter 1, patients' and service users' perceptions of service quality result from a comparison of their expectations before they receive the service to their actual experience of the service (Parasuraman *et al.* 1985). In order to monitor service quality it can therefore be useful to elicit information on both user expectations and their perceptions. Examples of how this can be done are given in Table 9.6. The idea is to get feedback both on what people expect from good service provision and how they perceive the particular service they received. For example, suppose two different patients circled the number 3 for their perceptions on whether they had a wide choice of meals, but in fact one of them wasn't particularly bothered about having such a choice, while having a wide range of choice was really important to the second one. The first patient may be quite happy about this aspect, while the second is clearly dissatisfied. By asking about expectations and perceptions, the real picture emerges, whereas if they were just asked about their perceptions we would not know whether they were satisfied.

An alternative to asking about expectations is to ask patients and service users to rate the importance to them of particular aspects of the service provided. For example, Belfast Maternity Hospital assessed service quality by issuing questionnaires to patients, their partners and staff. Staff were asked to answer the questions from the patients' perspective. Each group was asked to do two things (Hill and McCrory 1997):

- rate a wide variety of clinical and non-clinical service factors, using the scale 'very good', 'good', 'indifferent', 'poor' and 'very poor';

Table 9.7 Importance ratings and perceptions of mothers for certain service factors at Belfast Maternity Hospital

Service factor	% of mothers rating this factor 'very important' or 'important'	% of mothers rating the hospital 'very good' or 'good' on this factor
Communication between staff and patients	100	95
Cleanliness and hygiene	100	88
Appearance of delivery suite rooms	75	87
Quality of food	88	49
Car parking	84	51
Vending machines	34	17

- give an importance rating on each factor on the scale: 'very important', 'important', 'neither important nor unimportant', 'unimportant' or 'totally unimportant'.

Table 9.7 shows just a very small sample of the information collected, and in particular does *not* show the responses of partners and staff. However, it does illustrate very well the benefits of the hospital's approach. This example demonstrates clearly the benefits of asking about relative importance. Without the middle column, there is no systematic way of demonstrating that the priority for improvement in the hospital is *not* the vending machines!

Delivering excellence: a final word

Excellence in health and social care is something to which staff, service users, patients and carers all aspire. It is hoped that this book will contribute to helping service organizations move further on the road to excellence and deliver better quality services for people, many of whom will be feeling anxious and vulnerable.

There are a number of pointers for delivering excellence in health and social care. These include:

- Get to know your patients and service users. Find out about their experiences using your services and their ideas for improving them.
- Talk to your staff and colleagues about their ideas for improving services. What would help them do their jobs better?
- Use the Excellence Model, or something similar, if only to provide a baseline assessment of the strengths and weaknesses of your service or organization. Start with 'customer results'. How do they compare with what you and your service users would ideally like to see? Identify with staff, and if possible with user representatives, which of the enablers of the model need most attention to deliver better results for service users. Develop an action plan based on what you find out and implement it.
- Even if you don't wish to use the terms 'vision' and 'mission', write down what you see as the core objectives of your services and the core values that you aspire to. Translate these objectives into detailed policies and strategies, consistent with service values.
- Draw a process map or diagram showing how your processes work from the viewpoint of both users and staff. Identify which activities add value and which do not. Think creatively about ways to eliminate some of the activities that do not add value in order to speed up the process and reduce costs, while improving the service to users.

- Look at how patients and users access your service or how they are referred to your department or clinic. If they are referred by people outside your department, how well do these people understand your service and how well do you understand things from their viewpoint? Are there unnecessary delays or problems that occur? Do other professionals provide services to your service users, and if so do users receive a joined-up service? In each case communication and effective partnership working are vital.
- Visit similar units to your own in other geographical areas. Do they do things differently? What can you learn from them? Look at their performance measures and compare them with yours. What do they do better?
- Examine the performance measures currently used for your services. How well do they reflect the experience of your service users? Do they take account of the requirements of other key stakeholders?
- Be aware of the pitfalls of managing change in organizations. Make sure you carry the bulk of your staff with you. Do they feel that their concerns are listened to and taken into account?
- Give due attention to staff training and development. Make sure that staff are trained in service aspects of their job as well as their clinical or professional roles.
- Make sure that staff feel recognized and rewarded when they deliver good service. Aim to create enthusiasm and a climate of openness rather than a blame culture.

Finally, remember that in essence the approach to delivering excellence is not difficult. The following advice, based on TNT's 'Winning Formula', is a useful guide here:

- ask service users what they want;
- equip staff to satisfy service users and other key stakeholders;
- measure key outcomes for improvement;
- create enthusiasm and success;
- strive to beat previous best performance;
- provide recognition and always say thank you.

References

Abbott, L. (1955) *Quality and Competition*. Columbia, SC: Columbia University Press.

Adair, J. (1987) *Effective Teambuilding*, 2nd edn. London: Pan Books.

Adams, L. (1998) Measuring service quality in social services, *Management Issues in Social Care*, 3(5): 19–25.

Andersen, B. (1995) Benchmarking, in A. Rolstadas (ed.) *Performance Management: A Business Process Benchmarking Approach*, pp. 211–42. London: Chapman & Hall.

Anderson, D.N. (1988) *Quality: A Positive Business Strategy*. St Paul: 3M Quality Management Services.

Audit Commission (1997) *The Melody Lingers On: A Review of the Audits of People, Pay and Performance*. London: Audit Commission.

Audit Scotland (2001) *Managing People in the NHS in Scotland: Self-assessment Handbook*. Edinburgh: Audit Scotland.

Bemrose, C. and MacKeith, J. (1996) *Partnerships for Progress: Good Practice in the Relationship Between Local Government and Voluntary Organisations*. Bristol: The Policy Press.

Bennis, W. and Nanus, B. (1985) *Leaders: The Strategies for Taking Charge*. New York: Harper & Row.

Beresford, P. (2000) Service users' knowledge and social work theory: conflict or collaboration? *British Journal of Social Work*, 30(4): 489–503.

Berry, L. (1995) *On Great Service*. New York: The Free Press.

Berry, L., Zeithaml, V. and Parasuraman, A. (1985) *A Practical Approach to Quality*. New York: Joiner Associates Inc.

Berry, L., Zeithaml, V. and Parasuraman, A. (1988) The service quality puzzle, *Business Horizons*, Sept.–Oct.: 35–43.

Bevan, G. and Bawden, D. (2001) Clinical data and information, and clinical governance, *Clinical Governance Bulletin*, 2(2): 2–3.

Bevan, H. (1997) *24 Ways to Re-design your Healthcare Process*. Leicester: Leicester Royal Infirmary NHS Trust.

Bond, H. (1998) Bridging a gulf, *Community Care*, 10–16 September: 30–1.

Bounds, G.M., Yorks, L., Adams, M. and Ranney, G. (1994) *Beyond TQM: Toward the Emerging Paradigm*. New York: McGraw-Hill.

Bowen, D.E. and Lawler, E.E. III (1994) *Employee Empowerment in Service Firms: Answering the Growing Questions*, working paper. Quoted in L. Berry (1995) *On Great Service*. New York: The Free Press.

British Quality Association (1990) *Guidance on the Interpretation of BS5750 to Social Care Agencies*. London: BQA.

British Telecom (BT) (1991) *Guide to Prospective Shareholders*. London: BT.

Broh, R.A. (1982) *Managing Quality for Higher Profits*. New York: McGraw-Hill.

Burbach, F.R. and Quarry, A. (1991) Quality and outcome in a community mental health team, *International Journal of Health Care Quality Assurance*, 4(2): 18–26.

Cabinet Office (1999) *Assessing Excellence: A Guide to Using Self-assessment to Achieve Performance Improvement in the Public Sector*. London: Cabinet Office.

Caldwell, P. (1984) Cultivating human potential at Ford, *The Journal of Business Strategy*, spring: 75.

Capital Carers (1998) *The Caring Link to Quality Care in the Community*. London: Capital Carers.

Carers Advisory Group (2001) *The London Mental Health Carers' Charter: Working with Carers*. London: Carers Advisory Group.

Carlzon, J. (1987) *Moments of Truth*. Cambridge, MA: Ballinger.

Carr, D.K. and Littman, I.D. (1993) *Excellence in Government*. London: Coopers & Lybrand.

Carruthers, I. and Holland, P. (1991) Quality assurance: choice for the individual, *International Journal of Health Care Quality Assurance*, 4(2): 9–17.

Casson, S. and Johnson, M. (1996) *Total Quality in Services for Homeless Young People*. London: Centrepoint.

Casson, S. and Manning, B. (1997) *Total Quality in Child Protection: A Manager's Guide*. Lyme Regis: Russell House Publishing.

Casson, S., Robinson, D. and De Ste. Croix, R. (1997) Making the quality journey in home care, *CCMP*, 5(6): 202–8.

CIMA (1993) *Research Study: Performance Measurement in the Manufacturing Sector*. London: CIMA.

Conti, T. (1997) Optimising self-assessment, *Total Quality Management*, 8(2&3): S5–15.

Cook, S. (1992) *Customer Care: Implementing Total Quality in Today's Service-driven Organisation*. London: Kogan Page.

Copeland, G.P. (2001) Outcome analysis as a clinical governance tool: experiences with the POSSUM system, *Clinical Governance Bulletin*, 2(2): 4–5.

Couldstone, J. (1999) The makers of leaders, *UK Excellence*, February.

Coulson-Thomas, C. (ed.) (1994) *Business Process Re-engineering: Myth and Reality*. London: Kogan Page.

Crosby, P.B. (1984) *Quality Without Tears*. New York: McGraw-Hill.

Crosby, P.B. (1992) Does the Baldrige Award really work? *Harvard Business Review*, January/February: 127–8.

David, A.J. (1988) *The customer/supplier relationship*. Paper presented to the International Conference on TQM, June.

Deming, W.E. (1982) *Quality, Productivity and Competitive Position*. Cambridge, MA: Massachusetts Institute of Technology.

Deming, W.E. (1986) *Out of the Crisis*. Cambridge, MA: Massachusetts Institute of Technology.

Deming, W.E. (1993) *The New Economies*. Cambridge, MA: Massachusetts Institute of Technology.

Department of Health (DoH) (1997) *The New NHS: Modern, Dependable*, Cm 3807. London: The Stationery Office.

Department of Health (DoH) (1998a) *A First Class Service: Quality in the New NHS*. London: The Stationery Office.

Department of Health (DoH) (1998b) *Working Together: Securing a Quality Workforce for the NHS*. London: The Stationery Office.

Department of Health (DoH) (1998c) *Modernising Social Services*, Cm 4169. London: The Stationery Office.

Department of Health (DoH) (1998d) *The Quality Protects Programme: Transforming Children's Services*, LAC(98)28. London: The Stationery Office.

Department of Health (DoH) (1999a) *Patient and Public Involvement in the New NHS*. London: The Stationery Office.

Department of Health (DoH) (1999b) *Working Together to Safeguard Children*. London: The Stationery Office.

Department of Health (DoH) (1999c) *Caring about Carers: A National Strategy for Carers*. London: The Stationery Office.

Department of Health (DoH) (2000a) *An Organisation with a Memory*. London: The Stationery Office.

Department of Health (DoH) (2000b) *A Quality Strategy for Social Care*. London: The Stationery Office.

Department of Health (DoH) (2001a) *NHS Performance Indicators: A Consultation*. London: The Stationery Office.

Department of Health (DoH) (2001b) *Fostering Services: National Minimum Standards and Fostering Services Regulations Consultation Document*. London: The Stationery Office.

Department of the Environment, Transport and the Regions (DETR) (1998) *Modernising Local Government: Improving Local Services Through Best Value*. London: DETR.

Department of the Environment, Transport and the Regions (DETR) (1999) Local Government Act 1999: Part I, *Best Value*. London: DETR.

Department of Trade and Industry (DTI) (1990) *The Case for Costing Quality*. London: HMSO.

Dillon, A. (2001) NICE and Clinical Governance, in M. Lugon and J. Secker-Walker (eds) *Advancing Clinical Governance*, pp. 137–48. London: The Royal Society of Medicine Press.

Donabedian, A. (1980) *Explorations in Quality Assessment and Monitoring, Vol.1: The Definition of Quality and Approaches to its Assessment*. London: Health Administration Press.

Dotchin, J. (1994) *Key Methods: Distance Learning Pack for MSc TQM and Business Excellence*. Sheffield: Sheffield Hallam University.

EFQM (European Foundation for Quality Management) (1999) *The EFQM Excellence Model: Public and Voluntary Sectors*. Brussels: European Foundation for Quality Management.

Ernst & Young Quality Improvement Consulting Group (1992) *Total Quality*. London: Kogan Page.

Excellence North West (2000) *Guide to Organisational Excellence*. Bolton: Excellence North West.

Feigenbaum, A.V. (1991) *Total Quality Control*, 3rd edn. New York: McGraw-Hill.

Feinnman, J. (2001) Too much information? *Observer*, 11 November: 63.

Foggin, J.H. (1991) Closing the gaps in services marketing, in M.J. Stahl and G.M. Bounds (eds) *Competing Globally Through Customer Value*. New York: Quorum Books.

Freund, R.A. (1985) Definitions and basic quality concepts, *Journal of Quality Technology*, 17: 50–6.

Garvin, D.A. (1984) What does product quality really mean? *Sloan Management Review*, 26: 25–43.

Garvin, D.A. (1993) *On Knowledge Management*. Boston, MA: Harvard Business School Press.

Gaster, L. (1995) *Quality in Public Services*. Buckingham: Open University Press.

George, M. (2001) Quick thinking, *Guardian*, 5 December: 92.

Gilmore, H.L. (1974) Product conformance cost. *Quality Progress*, 7: 16–19.

Glanfield, P. (2001) *Towards Sustainable Change and Improvement*, working paper. Sheffield: Trent Regional Health Authority.

Goasdoue, J. (1990) quoted in Dept of Trade and Industry, *The Case for Costing Quality*. London: HMSO.

Goldratt, E. (1990) *Theory of Constraints*. Great Barrington, MA: North River Press.

Goldratt, E. and Cox, J. (1993) *The Goal: A Process of Ongoing Improvement*. Aldershot: Gower.

Gronroos, C. (1983) *Strategic Management and Marketing in the Service Sector*. Cambridge, MA: Marketing Science Institute.

Groocock, J.M. (1986) *The Chain of Quality*. New York: Wiley.

Gufreda, J., Maynard, L. and Lytle, L. (1992) Employee involvement in the quality process, in Ernst & Young Quality Improvement Consulting Group, *Total Quality: A Manager's Guide for the 1990s*. London: Kogan Page.

Haigh, B. and Morris, D.S. (2001) *Total Quality Management: A Case Study Approach*. Sheffield: Sheffield Hallam University Press.

Hammer, M. and Champy, J. (1993) *Re-engineering the Corporation: A Manifesto for Business Revolution*. London: Nicholas Brealey.

Harding, T. and Beresford, P. (1996) *The Standards We Expect*. London: National Institute for Social Work.

Hardy, B., Hudson, B. and Waddington, E. (2000) *What Makes a Good Partnership?* Leeds: Nuffield Institute for Health.

Harr, R. (2001) TQM in dental practice, *International Journal of Health Care Quality Assurance*, 14(2): 69–81.

Harrington, H.J. (1991) *Business Process Improvement*. New York: McGraw-Hill.

Haywood-Farmer, J. (1988) A conceptual model of service quality, *International Journal of Operations and Production Management*, 8(6): 19–29.

Hill, F.M. and McCrory, M.L. (1997) Measuring service quality at Belfast Maternity Hospital, *Total Quality Management*, 8(5): 229–42.

Hines, P. and Taylor, D. (2000) *Going Lean: A Guide to Implementation*. Cardiff: Lean Enterprise Research Centre, Cardiff University.

Hopson, B. and Scally, M. (1991) *12 Steps to Success Through Service*. London: Mercury Books.

Hughes, A.D. (1999) An investigation of self-assessment and the business excellence model using the teachings of Dr W. Edwards Deming. MSc Thesis in TQM, Sheffield Hallam University.

Humphrey, N. and Hildrew, M. (1992) Napier House: the steps to quality, *International Journal for Health Care Quality Assurance*, 5(3): 35–6.

Hutchings, D. (1990) *In Pursuit of Quality*. London: Pitman.

Iles, D.F. (1990) Missing reports in outpatients: a problem solved with quality assured, *International Journal of Health Care Quality Assurance*, 3(2): 25–9.

Iles, V. and Sutherland, K. (2001) *Organisational Change: A Review for Health Care Managers, Professionals and Researchers*. London: National Coordinating Centre for NHS Service Delivery and Organisation.

Imai, M. (1986) *Kaizen: The key to Japanese Competitive Success*. New York: Random House.

Institute of Directors (1997) *Business Excellence: A Director's Guide*. London: The Director Publications Ltd.

International Standards Organisation (2000) *ISO9001:2000 Quality Management Systems Requirements*. Geneva: ISO.

Joiner, B. and Scholtes, P.R. (1988) The manager's new job, in R.L. Chase (ed.) *TQM: An IFS Executive Briefing*. Bedford: IFS Publications.

Joseph Rowntree Foundation (2000) *Older People's Definitions of Quality Services*. York: Joseph Rowntree Foundation.

Joss, R. and Kogan, M. (1995) *Advancing Quality: Total Quality Management in the National Health Service*. Buckingham: Open University Press.

Judd, D.K. and Winder, R.E. (1995) The psychology of quality, *Total Quality Management*, 6(3).

Juran, J.M. (1986) The quality trilogy, *Quality Progress*, 19(8): 9–24.

Juran, J.M. (ed.) (1988) *Quality Control Handbook*. New York: McGraw-Hill.

Juran, J.M. (1989) *Juran on Leadership for Quality*. New York: The Free Press.

Kalter, T.L., Neilsen, C.C. and Psonak, R.A. (1989) Factors affecting the use of prosthetic services, *Journal of Prosthetics and Orthotics*, 1(4): 242–9.

Kanter, R. (1983) *The Change Masters*. New York: Simon & Schuster.

Kaplan, R.S. and Norton, D.P. (1992) The balanced scorecard: measures that drive performance, *Harvard Business Review*, 70(1): 71–9.

Kaplan, R.S. and Norton, D.P. (1996) *The Balanced Scorecard: Translating Strategy into Action*. Boston, MA: Harvard Business School Press.

Kennerley, M. and Neely, A. (2000) Performance measurement frameworks: a review. *Proceedings of Performance Measurement 2000: Past, Present and Future*, Robinson College, Cambridge, 19–21 July, pp. 291–8.

Kingston upon Hull City Council (1999) *Guide to the Quality Management System for Kingston upon Hull City Council*. Hull: Kingston upon Hull City Council.

Koch, H. (1991) *Total Quality Management in Health Care*. Harlow: Longman.

Kwong, C.S. (2001) Evaluation of the contribution of ISO9000 to the quality of prosthesis at the artificial limb centre of Tan Tock Seng Hospital, Singapore. MSc thesis in TQM and Business Excellence, Sheffield Hallam University.

Leffler, K.B. (1982) Ambiguous changes to product quality, *American Economic Review*, December: 41–52.

Levitt, T. (1972) Production-line approach to service, *Harvard Business Review*, 50(5): 41–52.

Lewis, F. (1984) The Tiffany model, *New York Times*, 7 June: 31.

Long, P.D. (1996) *Systems and Processes* (learning pack for the MSc in TQM and Business Excellence). Sheffield: Sheffield Hallam University.

Lowe, J.A. and McBean, G.M. (1989) Honesty without fear, *Proceedings of the 43rd Annual Congress of the American Society for Quality Control*. Toronto: American Society for Quality Control.

Lugon, M. and Secker-Walker, J. (2001) *Advancing Clinical Governance*. London: The Royal Society of Medicine Press.

Mann, N.R. (1985) *The Keys to Excellence: The Story of the Deming Philosophy*. Los Angeles: Prestwick Books.

Martensen, A. and Dahlgaard, J.J. (1999) Integrating business excellence and innovation management, *Total Quality Management*, 10(4&5): S627–35.

Martin, W.B. (1989) *Managing Quality Customer Service*. London: Kogan Page.

Maxwell, R. (1984) Quality assessment in health, *British Medical Journal*, 13: 31–4.

McNeish, D. (1999) Promoting participation for children and young people: some key questions for health and social welfare organisations, *Journal of Social Work Practice*, 13(2): 191–203.

McSweeney, P. (1997) Quality in primary care: management challenges for new health authorities, *Total Quality Management*, 8(5): 243–53.

Midgley, S. (2001) Banking on cooperation, *NHS Magazine*, 2(3): 22–3.

Modernisation Agency (2001) *The Modernisation Agency*. London: Modernisation Agency.

Moullin, M. (1995) Getting across the quality message, in G.K. Kanji (ed.) *Total Quality Management: Proceedings of the First World Congress*, pp. 612–15. London: Chapman & Hall.

Moullin, M. (1997) Quality: the experts' view. Presentation to the 2nd World Congress for TQM, Sheffield.

Moullin, M. (1999) *Managing Quality: Managing Service Delivery*, Book 3. Milton Keynes: The Open University.

Moullin, M. (2002) Using the performance prism to evaluate a health service taskforce. Paper presented to the European Academy of Management Annual Conference EURAM, Stockholm, May.

Munchi, K.F. (1992) Averting a reversal of TQM, in *Transactions of the ASQC Quality Congress*. Nashville, TN: American Society for Quality Control.

Murphy, J.A. (1993) Inverting the pyramid, *European Quality*, special showcase edition, June: 78–82.

National Health Service (NHS) (2000) *The NHS Plan*, Cm 4818-I. London: HMSO.

National Institute for Social Work (NISW) (1999) *Standards of Practice for Social Work and Social Care: Towards a Consistent Quality Service – NISW Briefing no. 25*. London: NISW.

National Institute for Social Work (NISW) (2000) *Modernising Social Work – NISW Briefing no. 29*. London: NISW.

National Institute for Social Work (NISW) (2001) *Putting the Person First – NISW Briefing no. 31*. London: NISW.

National Primary Care Development Team (2002) *PDSA Basics*. www.npdt.org/res/pdsa.htm (accessed January 2002).

National Schizophrenia Fellowship (NSF) (2001) *Commitment to Carers*. London: NSF.

Neely, A. (1998) *Measuring Business Performance*. London: Profile Books.

Neely, A., Adams, C. and Crowe, P. (2001) The performance prism in practice, *Measuring Business Excellence*, 5(2): 6–13.

Neely, A. and Bourne M. (2000) Why measurement initiatives fail, *Measuring Business Excellence*, 4(4): 3–6.

Neilsen, C.C. (1991) A survey of amputees: functional level and life satisfaction, information needs and the prosthetist's role, *Journal of Prosthetics and Orthotics*, 3(3): 125–9.

NHS Executive (1999a) *Clinical Governance: Quality in the New NHS*. Wetherby: Department of Health.

NHS Executive (1999b) *The NHS Performance Assessment Framework*. Wetherby: Department of Health.

NHS Executive Trent (2001) *Modernising the NHS in Trent: Trent Improvement Network*. www.nhsetrent.gov.uk/modernisation/tim.htm (accessed 2001).

Nicholls, S., Cullen, R. and Halligan, A. (2001) Using clinical information: measurement, *Clinical Governance Bulletin*, 2(2): 7–9.

Normann, R. *et al.* (1978) *Development Strategies for Swedish Service Knowledge* (in Swedish). Stockholm: SIAR.

Northern and Yorkshire NHS Modernisation Programme (2001) *Mental Health Improving Practice*. www.nyx.org.uk/modernprogrammes/mentalhealth (accessed 27 Nov. 2001).

Nwabuese, U. and Kanji, G.K. (1997) The implementation of total quality management in the NHS: how to avoid failure, *Total Quality Management*, 8(5): 265–80.

Oakland, J.S. (1995) *Total Quality Management*. Oxford: Butterworth Heinemann.

Oakland, J.S. (1999) *Total Organizational Excellence*. Oxford: Butterworth Heinemann.

Oakland, J.S. (2000) *Total Quality Management: Text with Cases*, 2nd edn. Oxford: Butterworth Heinemann.

Osman, A. (1996) ISO certification: the key to sustainable competitive advantage, in B. Whitford and R. Bird (eds) *The Pursuit of Quality*. London: Prentice Hall.

Øvretveit, J. (1990) What is quality in health services? *Health Services Management*, June: 132–3.

Øvretveit, J. (1997) Learning from quality improvement in Europe and beyond, *Journal of the Joint Commission for Accreditation of Healthcare Organisations*, 23(1): 7–22.

Painter, A. and Johnson, G. (1997) *The Use of the EFQM Model of Business Excellence as a Framework for Cultural and Organisational Change in Cheshire Social Services*. Chester: Cheshire County Council.

Parasuraman, A., Zeithaml, V. and Berry, L. (1985) A conceptual model of service quality and its implications for future research, *Journal of Marketing*, 49(Autumn): 41–50.

Pavlou, P.G. and Chisnell, C.A. (1997) European Business Excellence Model: implementation experiences of the Salford Royal Hospitals NHS Trust. *Human Resources in the NHS*, 14(6): 2–3.

Peters, T.J. and Austin, N. (1985) *A Passion for Excellence*. New York: Random House.

Pettigrew, A. (1998) Success and failure in corporate transformation initiatives, in R.D. Galliers and W.R.J. Baets (eds) *Information Technology and Organisational Transformation*. Chichester: Wiley.

Pfeffer, N. and Coote, A. (1991) *Is Quality Good for You? A Critical Review of Quality Assurance in Welfare Services*. London: Institute for Public Policy Research.

Philips (1986) *Involvement in Quality: Some Philips Experiences*. Eindhoven: Philips.

Phipps, B. (1999) Hitting the bottleneck, *Health Management*, February: 16–17.

Pirsig, R.M. (1974) *Zen and the Art of Motorcycle Maintenance*. New York: Bantam.

Praxiom (2001) ISO9001:2000. http://praxiom.com/iso-9001-standard.html (accessed 7 Sept. 2001).

Pringle, M. (2001) *Response to Speech by Sir Donald Irvine. Royal College of General Practitioners Press Release*, 16 January. London: RCGP.

Quality Standards Task Group (1998) *Quality Standards in the Voluntary Sector*. London: Quality Standards Task Group.

Quality Standards Task Group (2001) *Excellence in View: Case Studies Using the Excellence Model*. London: Quality Standards Task Group.

Rajan, A. and Van Eupen, P. (1996) *Leading People*. London: Create/CILNTEC.

Reeves, C.A. and Bednar, D.A. (1994) Defining quality: alternatives and implications, *Academy of Management Review*, 19(3): 419–45.

Robbins, H. and Finley, M. (1996) *Why Teams Don't Work*. London: Orion Business.

Ross, J.E. (1994) *TQM: Text, Cases and Readings*, 2nd edn. London: Kogan Page.

Scholtes, P.R. (1998) *The Leader's Handbook*. New York: McGraw-Hill.

Scholtes, P.R. (1999) The new Competencies of Leadership, *Total Quality Management*, 10(4&5): S704–10.

Scottish Office/COSLA (1997) *Best Value in Local Government: Report of the Joint Scottish Office/Convention of Scottish Local Authorities Best Value Task Force*. Edinburgh: Scottish Office.

Scottish Office Social Work Services Group (1998) *Hospital Discharge for Frail Older People*. London: HMSO.

Senge, P.M. (1990) *The Fifth Discipline: the Art and Practice of the Learning Organisation*. Cambridge, MA: Harvard University Press.

Senge, P.M. (1992) *The Fifth Discipline*. London: Century Business.

Shergold, K. and Reed, D.M. (1996) Striving for excellence: how self-assessment using the Business Excellence Model can result in step improvements in all areas of business activities, *The TQM Magazine*, 8(6): 48–52.

Shewhart, W.A. (1931) *Economic Control of Quality of a Manufactured Product*. New York: Van Nostrand.

Smith, G. (1998) Three HR issues affecting social care, *Management Issues in Social Care*, 5(3): 27–9.

Smith, G.F. (1993) The meaning of quality, *Total Quality Management*, 4(3): 235–44.

Stahr, H., Bulman, B. and Stead, M. (2000) *The Excellence Model in the Health Sector: Sharing Good Practice*. Chichester: Kingsham Press.

Staines, A. (2000) Benefits of an ISO9001 certification: the case of a Swiss regional hospital, *International Journal of Health Care Quality Assurance*, 13(1): 952–6862.

Stebbing, L. (1990) *Quality Management in the Service Industry*. Chichester: Ellis Horwood.

Taguchi, G. (1986) *Introduction to Quality Engineering*. Tokyo: Asian Productivity Organisation.

Talwar, R. (1994) Re-engineering: a wonder drug for the 90s? in C. Coulson-Thomas (ed.) *Business Process Re-engineering: Myth and Reality*. London: Kogan Page.

Taylor, D. (2001) *Business Excellence in the Health Service, Business Standards, December 2000/January 2001*. London: British Standards Institute.

Thomas, B. (1994) *The Human Dimension of Quality*. London: McGraw-Hill.

Toon, P. (1994) *What is Good General Practice?* London: RCGP.

Torres, O.U. (1997) Measuring service quality in a children's hospital. MSc thesis, Sheffield Hallam University.

Trapp, R. (1997) Where have all the leaders gone? in Institute of Directors, *Business Excellence: A Director's Guide*. London: The Director Publications Ltd.

Triseliotis, J., Sellick, C. and Short, R. (1995) *Foster Care: Theory and Practice*. London: Batsford.

Tucker, A. (2001) in J. Feinnman, Life and soul: handle with care, *Observer*, 25 November.

Van Gigch, J.P. (1977) Quality: producer and consumer views, *Quality Progress*, April.

Vroom, V.H. and Yago, A.G. (1988) *The New Leadership: Managing Participation in Organisations*. Hemel Hempstead: Prentice Hall.

Wellins, R.S., Byham, W.C. and Wilson, J.M. (1991) *Empowered Teams*. San Francisco: Jossey-Bass.

Wiffen, J. (2001) Beyond listening: involving children, young people and their families in the planning of children's services. Talk to British Quality Foundation Social Care Networking Group, London.

Womack, J. and Jones, D. (1996) *Lean Thinking: Banish Waste and Create Wealth in your Corporation*. New York: Simon & Schuster.

Zeithaml, V., Parasuraman, A. and Berry, L. (1990) *Delivering Quality Service*. New York: The Free Press.

Index

Page numbers in *italics* refer to figures and tables.